The Clueless
Vegetarian

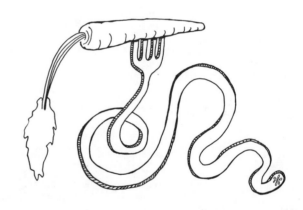

The Clueless Vegetarian

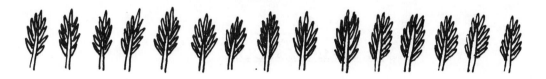

A Cookbook for the Aspiring Vegetarian

EVELYN RAAB

FIREFLY BOOKS

For my husband, George, and my sons, Dustin and Jared, who patiently endured more than a few extraordinarily weird meals during the writing of this book. Thank you for your support and encouragement—and thank you for being brave enough to taste everything at least once. I promise never to make that—you know what—ever again.

Acknowledgements

Thank you to Brenda Wines-Moher, RD, and Caroline Doris, RD, at the Peterborough County City Health Unit for their help with the nutritional information in this book.

A big thank you to Celia Hunter whose meticulous proofreading helped avert innumerable embarrassing and ridiculous typo-related recipe disasters.

A special thanks to all my friends (you know who you are) who have allowed me to borrow some of their favorite recipes to include in *The Clueless Vegetarian*.

And thanks, Mom—you taught me to treat vegetables with the utmost respect. Your cabbage noodles are legendary.

A FIREFLY BOOK

A Firefly Book

Copyright © 2000 by Evelyn Raab
Illustration copyright © 2000 by George Walker

U.S. Cataloguing-in-Publication Data

Evelyn, Raab.
    The clueless vegetarian / Evelyn Raab.—1st ed.
[216]p. : ill. ; cm.
Includes index.
Summary: Includes nutritional information, ideas for creating recipes, and simple recipes for all types of foods.
ISBN 1-55209-497-9 (pbk)
1. Vegetarian cookery. 2. Cookery—Vegetables. I. Title.
641.5/ 636 —21   2000   CIP

Published in the United States in 2000
by Firefly Books (U.S.) Inc.
P.O. Box 1338
Ellicott Station
Buffalo, New York, USA
14205

First published in Canada in 2000 by Key Porter Books Limited

Electronic formatting: Jean Lightfoot Peters

Printed and bound in Canada

introduction

So you're a vegetarian. Or you're thinking about it. Or you live with a vegetarian. Or perhaps you just have to feed one occasionally.

But you don't want to eat only weird food. Or spend all day cooking it.

Congratulations. You've come to the right place.

The Clueless Vegetarian is designed for vegetarians who love good food, cooked from scratch, but who also want to have a life. This book is filled with simple recipes for just about anything you might ever want to eat, and a few things you wouldn't touch with a ten-foot pole. You'll find recipes for lasagne, chili and burritos. There are curries and casseroles. There are hearty soups and satisfying snacks. And even some truly decadent desserts.

There are, of course, also recipes using tofu, tempeh and texturized vegetable protein. Because you do have to know about this stuff. Really.

If you're just switching to a vegetarian diet, *The Clueless Vegetarian* gives you the straightforward nutritional information you need to help you make good food choices (without obsessing). There are hints for concocting vegetarian versions of your favorite old recipes, and suggestions on preparing meals for the mixed household. You'll even find cooking advice and survival tips that are just plain useful for anyone, vegetarian or not.

Now, let's start with the basics, shall we? We'll save the tempeh for later. It's best to work up to these things gradually.

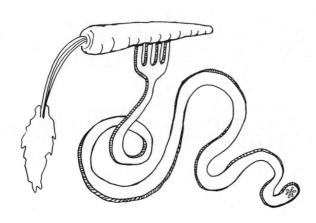

Contents

Icons Used in This Book 8

1. Vegetarian Survival Skills 9

What Kind of Vegetarian Are You, Anyway? 10
Living Vegetarianly—Some Helpful Hints 11
The Vegetarian Food Guide 12
The Big Four: Vegetarian Nutrition in a Nutshell 14
How to Eat Out 17
Essential Supplies for the Vegetarian Kitchen 18
How to Vegetarianize a Recipe 20

2. Appetizers, Snacks and Starters 22

3. Soups from Scratch 38

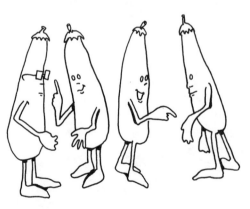

4. Serious Salads and Dynamic Dressings   56

5. Exceptional Eggs and Perfect Pancakes   83

6. Marvelous Main Dishes   94

Pastas and Sauces   95
Stir-fry Crazy   117
Chilis, Curries, Casseroles and Concoctions   126
Deeply Personal Pizzas   152
Random Delights   156

7. Sidekicks   167

Good Old Grains   168
Vegetables on the Side   178

8. Baked Stuff   186

9. Just Desserts   198

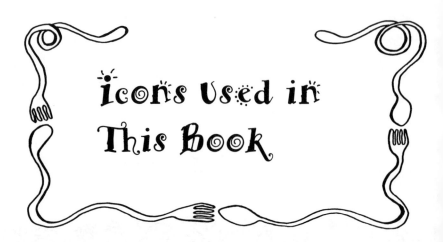

Icons Used in This Book

The following icons are used to identify the different sorts of recipes. A recipe may have more than one icon, meaning that it falls into many categories—for example, the recipe could contain both eggs and dairy and can be thrown together in 30 minutes or less.

 The recipe contains dairy ingredients, such as milk, cheese or yogurt.

 The recipe contains eggs.

 Vegan recipe. This means that the recipe is *entirely* vegan (no eggs or dairy products), or that it can be prepared as a vegan dish by omitting any optional eggs or dairy ingredients. If a recipe is identified with both dairy and vegan, it means that dairy ingredients are used in the dish, but reasonable vegan substitutions are suggested.

 Quick Fix! A recipe that can be thrown together from scratch in 30 minutes or less!

1. Vegetarian Survival Skills

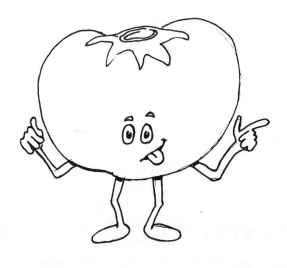

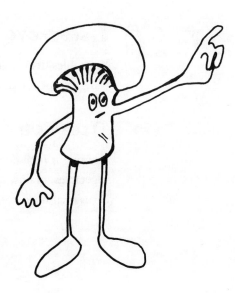

What Kind of Vegetarian Are You, Anyway?

There's more than one way to be a vegetarian. The choice you make depends, of course, on your moral convictions, your sense of spirituality and your cosmic connection to the totality of the universe. It also depends on what you like to eat and what sort of diet you're prepared to follow.

Vegan

Vegetables, fruits and grains only. That's it. Nothing that has ever had anything to do with any sort of living creature. Not even honey.

Ovo-vegetarian

Vegetables, fruits, grains and eggs.

Lacto-vegetarian

Vegetables, fruits, grains and dairy products. Products such as milk, cheese, yogurt and butter.

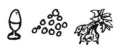

Lacto-ovo vegetarian

Vegetables, fruits, grains, eggs and dairy products. So, basically anything except actual meat, chicken or fish.

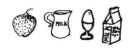

Occasional vegetarian

You might include chicken and/or fish in your diet (in addition to vegetables, grains, eggs and dairy products) or simply indulge in the occasional burger without feeling too guilty about it.

Living Vegetarianly— Some Helpful Hints

Eat a wide variety of foods. If you are finicky, creeped out by unfamiliar flavors or squeamish about trying new things, this is the time to get over it. While a vegetarian diet doesn't have to be a non-stop exotic adventure, you'll be missing a lot if you don't take full advantage of all the wonderful vegetarian foods that are out there.

Whenever possible choose whole, unrefined foods. Buy fresh fruits and vegetables in season, unprocessed cheeses, whole grain breads. The less someone else has fiddled around with your food, the better.

Make your calories count. If you're going to squander extra calories on something, wouldn't you rather it be something wonderful (like a fabulous dessert or some decadently delicious pasta) than a bag of simulated salt and vinegar potato chips?

If you've been invited to someone's home for dinner, let them know beforehand that you are a vegetarian and what, *exactly*, you will eat. This is no time to be shy. Your host/hostess will appreciate you being straightforward about this. Really. You might even offer to bring a vegetarian dish to share—thus guaranteeing that there will be at least one thing you can eat.

Teach your friends and family how to make vegetarian versions of familiar foods. Show them how to use tofu or tempeh in a stir-fry instead of meat, let them taste your veggie burrito, invite them to your home for a completely non-weird vegetarian meal. They'll never even miss the meat.

When you're planning a meal, stop thinking meat, potato and two vegetables. Instead, make a dinner out of several side dishes. Create a meal with soup as the centerpiece, accompanied by some good bread, a salad and a couple of appetizers. Or better yet, do *all* appetizers. After all, who doesn't love to nibble?

The Vegetarian Food Guide

This basic guide can help you determine whether your diet is on the right track. There is enough flexibility built into it to allow for the little personal idiosyncrasies (maybe you hate yogurt but you love lentils) that make each of us so wonderfully unique.

Grain Products
5–12 servings per day

Vegetables & Fruits
5–10 servings per day

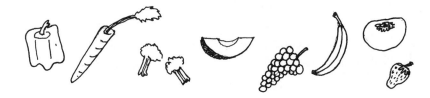

Beans & Eggs
2–4 servings per day

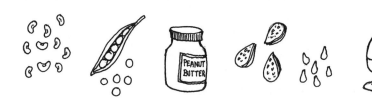

Milk & Milk Alteratives
4–6 servings per day

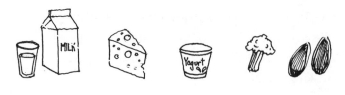

This food guide is an outline of your complete dietary require-ments for a single day. However, you don't have to fit every single food group into every single meal. Instead, take into consideration your eating habits over the course of the whole day—including snacks. Does the idea of 12 servings of grain products sound outrageous? It's not. Just one cup (250 mL) of pasta counts as two servings, and a whole bagel is another two—you're almost there already.

This guide is designed for a healthy, average adult. Children, pregnant or lactating women, and teens should consult a doctor or nutritionist for more specific guidelines.

Grain Products—5 to 12 servings per day
Bread, cereal, rice and pasta
One serving = 1 slice bread or ½ bagel or ½ cup (125 mL) pasta or rice or 2 crackers or 1 muffin

Vegetables and Fruits—5 to 10 servings per day
Fresh, frozen or canned vegetables, or fruit juice
One serving = 1 medium whole fruit or vegetable (like carrot, potato, apple, orange, banana) or ½ cup (125 mL) unsweetened fruit or veg-etable juice or 1 cup (250 mL) salad

Bean Products and Eggs—2 to 4 servings per day
Beans, soy products (like tofu or tempeh), nuts, seeds and eggs
One serving = ½ cup (125 mL) cooked beans or lentils or tofu or tempeh or 1 cup (250 mL) soy milk or 3 tbsp. (45 mL) peanut butter or 1 egg

Milk and Milk Alternatives—4 to 6 servings per day
Milk, yogurt and cheese (for those who use dairy products) or calcium-rich greens, almonds and tahini, and tofu made with calcium
One serving = ½ to 1 cup (125 mL to 250 mL) milk or yogurt or 1 ounce (28 g) cheese or 1 cup (250 mL) greens or ⅓ cup (75 mL) almonds or ½ cup (125 mL) tofu

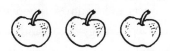

The Big Four: Vegetarian Nutrition in a Nutshell

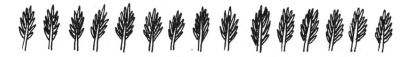

Okay, so you decide to become a vegetarian. You have your reasons. Fine. No one (except possibly your Aunt Gertrude) would dare argue with you about such things as your moral convictions regarding the sanctity of life or your belief in the spiritual oneness of the universe. But when it comes to the nutritional aspects of your vegetarian diet, you'd darn well better know what you're doing. It isn't hard. It just takes a little planning.

Now, a healthy lacto-ovo vegetarian diet is not only quite reasonable, but also fairly easy to follow. Nutritionally speaking, the main issues are protein, iron, vitamin B-12 and calcium. These are the Big Four. These are what Aunt Gertrude is concerned about. And, frankly, you should be too. Here's what you need to know (in a nutshell—okay, a coconut shell):

1. Protein—essential for growth, tissue repair and to help fight against infection

This is the biggie, isn't it? How (on earth) will you (ever) get enough protein if you're not eating meat (for goodness' sake, dear)? Well, it just so happens that meat isn't the only food that contains protein. A *responsible* (key word!) lacto-ovo vegetarian should have no problem obtaining adequate protein from a diet that includes a wide variety of foods—eggs, dairy products and legumes. If you are consuming enough calories to meet your energy needs, and assuming you do not depend *solely* on high-fat dairy products as your protein source, you can relax and eat your bean sprouts in peace. And furthermore, don't obsess over combining complementary proteins (beans and rice, for example) at the same meal. Instead, look at your total diet over the course of a whole day. Some whole wheat toast at breakfast, a bean salad at lunch, a slice of cheese, a scrambled egg, a little tofu—and you're doing just fine (thank you very much, Aunt Gertrude).

- Legumes (beans, peas and lentils)
- Soy foods (soybeans, tofu, tempeh, soy milk products)
- Peanut butter
- Seitan (wheat gluten)
- Nuts and seeds
- Grain products (wheat, rice, corn, barley, oats, millet, quinoa)
- Dairy products (milk, cheese, yogurt)
- Eggs

2. Iron—important for the formation of red blood cells

Plant foods (and also eggs) contain a different type of iron than red meat. It's *there*, it's just a bit harder to get at than the iron from red meats. In fact, vegetarian diets are often *higher* in total iron content than non-vegetarian diets, but the type of iron found in plant-based foods is poorly absorbed by the body. One thing that helps the body absorb this iron, however, is vitamin C. And that's the good news. Because a vegetarian diet tends to have plenty of vitamin C, it helps to unlock iron and make it available to the body. What does this mean to you? It means that you should choose foods that are a good source of iron, and make sure you're getting plenty of vitamin C as well. If all else fails, have a tall glass of orange juice with your oatmeal.

- Eggs
- Whole grains
- Dark green vegetables (broccoli, kale, peas, string beans, chard)
- Legumes (beans, lentils)
- Soy foods (soybeans, tofu, tempeh, soy milk products)
- Nuts and seeds (especially tahini and almond butter)
- Dried fruits (raisins, apricots, figs)
- Blackstrap molasses

3. B-12—needed for the formation of red blood cells and a healthy nervous system

Zinc—which can be found in chick-peas and lentils, as well as other legumes, sesame seeds, nuts, firm tofu, peanuts, wheat germ, milk products and eggs.

Vitamin D—available in fortified milk products, eggs and (yippee!) sunlight. So go outside once in a while.

Riboflavin—found in milk and eggs, as well as soybeans, almonds, enriched cereals and nutritional yeast. Also, oddly, mushrooms and sweet potatoes. Not to mention green leafy vegetables, dried fruits and whole grain products.

A healthy lacto-ovo vegetarian diet—one which includes dairy products and eggs—will usually provide adequate amounts of B-12. Since this nutrient is primarily found in animal products, only vegans need to make a special effort to obtain B-12 from alternative sources, such as fortified meat or egg substitutes (if available), or by using Red Star™ nutritional yeast, which can be sprinkled on salads, cooked grains or even on popcorn. It is also recommended that vegans have their blood levels of vitamin B-12 checked annually by a physician to see if any additional supplements are necessary.

- Dairy products (milk, cheese, yogurt)
- Fortified soy milk (if available)
- Fortified cereals
- Nutritional yeast (Red Star™ brand in particular)

4. Calcium—essential for teeth, bones and healthy muscle function

Calcium? No problem. If you're a lacto-ovo vegetarian, and you include dairy products in your diet, you should be laughing, calcium-wise. Milk, cheese and yogurt practically *scream* calcium. And if you also eat plenty of dark green vegetables (and why wouldn't you?) and some tofu or fortified soy milk and nibble the odd almond once in a while, you will be getting enough calcium. Post-menopausal women who aren't absolutely sure they're obtaining enough calcium from food are advised to take supplements to avoid osteoporosis.

- Dairy products (milk, cheese, yogurt)
- Fortified soy milk
- Fortified orange juice
- Dark green vegetables (broccoli, kale, collard greens)
- Dried figs
- Almonds
- Blackstrap molasses
- Legumes (beans and lentils)
- Soy foods (especially tofu made with calcium)

How To Eat Out

You really hate to make a spectacle of yourself. But for a vegetarian, eating out at a restaurant presents a challenge. Fortunately, there are more vegetarian choices on restaurant menus now than ever before, so it may not be so difficult to find something you can eat. Now take a deep breath, and have a close look at the menu. How about:

- Pizza (easy one).

- Pasta with veggie or cream sauce, or tossed with cheese.

- Veggie burgers or falafel.

- A bagel with cream cheese and a salad or an egg salad plate.

- Bean burritos or tacos (ask if the refried beans are made with vegetable shortening).

- Veggie or cheese submarine sandwich, just double the cheese and leave out the meat.

- Order a baked potato (or two) with vegetarian toppings.

- Have a huge salad, some good bread and dessert! (Watch out for bacon in a Caesar salad, or anchovies.)

- Go Indian—always lots of vegetarian choices.

- Try Chinese—but ask if there's any meat or fish. Remember, many Chinese dishes contain oyster sauce or chicken stock. Go for tofu or vegetable dishes and plain steamed rice. Soups are very often chicken-based.

- Make dinner out of appetizers—bruschetta, rice-stuffed grape leaves, veggie nachos with guacamole, fried zucchini sticks with dip, stuffed potato skins, antipasto without meat.

- Eat at a kosher dairy restaurant.

Essential Supplies for the Vegetarian Kitchen

Okay, so this is a wish list. You won't have all these things in your home all the time. Or even half the time. But let's say you did. Well, then, you could make almost everything in this book at a moment's notice. Now, wouldn't that be nice?

The Top Ten

If you were planning to get stranded on a desert island with nothing but a bathing suit, a can opener and ten food items, here's what you should pack. Oh, and by the way, don't forget your sunscreen.

- Rice
- Pasta
- Vegetable or olive oil
- Canned beans
- Tofu
- Peanut butter
- Canned tomatoes
- Onions
- Soy sauce
- Uh...chocolate (hey—you'll need *something*)

Pantry Staples

Canned and dry beans—several kinds (red kidney, black beans, chick-peas, white kidney, pinto)
Canned tomatoes
Canned spaghetti sauce (the best you can afford)
Vegetable oil (canola or sunflower)
Olive oil (yes, yes, yes)
Vinegar (wine or apple cider)
Balsamic vinegar
Soy sauce
Sesame oil
Peanut butter
Vegetable bouillon cubes or powder
Several kinds of pasta
Rice—white and brown
Cornmeal
Couscous
Bulghur wheat
Rolled oats

TVP (texturized vegetable protein)
Flour—white and whole wheat
Cornstarch
Raisins
Sun-dried tomatoes
Bread crumbs
Peanuts
Almonds
Walnuts
Pine nuts
Sesame seeds

Spices

Salt
Pepper
Oregano
Basil
Cumin
Turmeric
Curry powder
Cayenne
Crushed red pepper flakes
Cinnamon
Garam masala

Fresh Stuff

Tofu (regular and/or extra firm)
Eggs
Milk
Yogurt
Onions
Garlic
Potatoes
Fresh parsley
Cabbage
Carrots
Green and/or red peppers
Mushrooms
Broccoli
Eggplant

Lettuce (romaine, iceberg, leaf
    lettuce, mixed baby greens)
Green beans
Squash
Zucchini
Breads (several kinds—sandwich
    bread, tortillas, pita, bagels)
Cheeses (like Parmesan,
    Cheddar, mozzarella,
    Monterey Jack, Swiss, feta)

And in the freezer

Frozen peas
Frozen corn

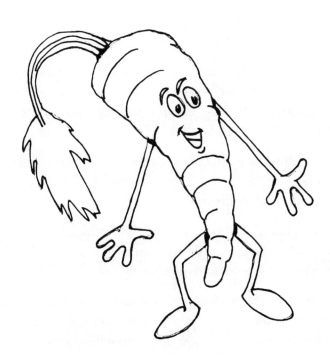

How to Vegetarianize a Recipe

Now look, no one would suggest that it is possible to create a vegetarian version of, say, roast beef. Although, no doubt, people have tried. However, in many cases you can create wonderful vegetarian versions of your old meat-based favorites. Or even adapt a new non-vegetarian recipe that you want to try by substituting something vegetarian for the meat. Here are a few hints to get you started:

★ Identify the problematic components in the recipe. Is meat the lead player, or does it just have a supporting role? Attempting to reproduce something like roast beef, for instance, is a desperate and often disappointing endeavor. However, if the meat plays a secondary role to any vegetables or sauce, you may be able to retain the integrity of the dish just by juggling ingredients.

★ A flavorful vegetable broth can almost always be used in place of beef or chicken broth in a recipe.

★ Instead of ground beef, substitute a similar volume of rehydrated TVP (texturized vegetable protein), frozen and defrosted tofu or mashed tempeh. Increase the other flavorings in the dish to compensate for the relative blandness of the meat stand-ins.

★ Try the chunk form of TVP (looks like dog kibble) instead of chunks of chicken or beef in stewy concoctions. Or use cubes of steamed tempeh or firm tofu.

★ Seitan (wheat gluten) can be used in place of sliced meat in a stir-fry or sauced dish. It has the right texture, anyway, and blends unobtrusively into whatever else is going on.

★ It may be possible to eliminate the meat from a dish altogether, without any adjustment. Or you can often just increase the amount of vegetables to make up for the missing meat.

★ Try eggplant or mushrooms instead of meat. Either one can provide a spongy, squishy texture that will more than compensate for whatever you took out.

★ Beans or lentils have a meaty quality that can add that certain something to a vegetarian dish. And bulgur wheat or cooked brown rice can provide a nice chewy texture.

★ Vegans can replace milk with soy milk with practically no difference in the final product. Soy cheese can sometimes take the place of regular cheese as well (but success will vary with the type of product—experiment).

★ If all else fails, try imitation meat. These products, made to resemble ground beef, pepperoni, hot dogs or hamburgers are widely available and will do the job when you're really feeling deprived.

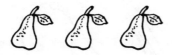

2. Appetizers, Snacks and Starters

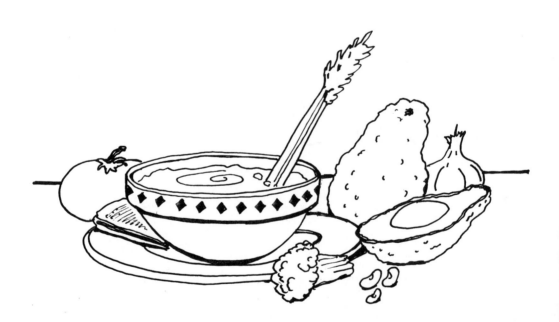

Hummus

This is the genuine article. Ridiculously easy. Why would you ever buy it ready-made? Try this stuffed into a pita pocket with some mixed greens and a shredded carrot.

1		(19-oz./540 mL) can chick-peas, drained but save the liquid (2 cups/500 mL home-cooked)
¼ cup	50 mL	tahini or, if unavailable, peanut butter
¼ cup	50 mL	lemon juice
2		cloves garlic, crushed
½ tsp.	2 mL	ground cumin
		salt and pepper to taste
		chopped parsley and olive oil for garnish (optional)

Measure all the ingredients, except the garnish, into the container of a blender or food processor, and blend until the mixture is very smooth, scraping down the sides 2 or 3 times. Taste and adjust the seasoning, if necessary. Hummus should be a little thicker than sour cream. If it's too thick, add a spoonful or two of the reserved liquid from the can of chick-peas and blend again.

To serve, spread the hummus out onto a platter, sprinkle with a little chopped parsley and drizzle the top with a bit of olive oil. Serve with triangles of warmed pita bread for dipping.

Makes about 2 cups (500 mL).

Tahini

Tahini is the Middle Eastern version of peanut butter. But instead of being used as a sandwich spread, tahini is a multipurpose ingredient that may be thinned and used as a sauce, or added to another dish as a flavoring. In some recipes it may be possible to use peanut butter instead (but the flavor will be different). Tahini is available in Middle Eastern grocery stores, and most large supermarkets.

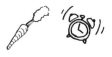

Chunky Avocado Salsa

No matter how much of this you make, you won't have enough.

2		large ripe avocados
1		small red onion, finely chopped
2 tbsp.	30 mL	lime juice
1		medium tomato, seeded and finely chopped
1		fresh jalapeño pepper, seeded and finely chopped
1 tsp.	5 mL	ground cumin
¼ cup	50 mL	chopped cilantro
½ tsp.	2 mL	salt

Cut the avocados in half, remove the pit and peel them. If they are ripe, the peel should come off easily. Dice the avocado flesh, and dump it into a bowl. Add all the remaining ingredients, and toss to combine without mashing. The ingredients should remain separate, and the salsa chunky.

Serve with tortilla chips for dipping, or as an accompaniment to tacos or burritos.

Makes about 2 cups (500 mL).

Avocado

Most avocados are picked while they're still unripe and only begin to soften once they're off the tree. Like in your kitchen, for instance. Just leave a hard avocado at room temperature until it yields to pressure when you (very, very gently) squeeze it in your hand. You can try to hurry this process by placing it in a paper bag with an apple. The apple will emit a gas (really) that helps other fruit to ripen. But whatever you do, don't refrigerate it before it's soft or it will never ripen properly.

SPECIAL BONUS PROJECT!

A Beautiful Avocado Plant for (Almost) Free

No! Stop! Don't throw out that avocado pit! It would be like, well, murder. Let it grow into a plant instead. Here's how you do it.

First, peel off as much of the brown outer skin as can easily be removed from the pit. Now, determine which end is up. (The bottom of the pit will be flatter, the top will be more pointy.) Next, poke three toothpicks around the "equator" of the pit, roughly equidistant from each other. Use these toothpicks to support the pit (bottom-side-down) over the opening of a wide-mouthed jar (like an old mayonnaise or jam jar). Fill the jar with enough water to come about halfway up the sides of the avocado pit, at least to the level of the toothpicks, and place it in a sunny spot. Now wait. For how long? Who knows? Probably weeks. Be patient.

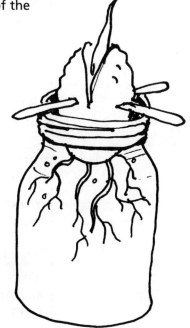

The first thing you will see is a root, sprouting out from the bottom of the pit. It will reach down into the water. Then, eventually, a shoot will appear at the top, then some leaves. At this point, you can plant it into a flowerpot filled with potting soil. Keep it on a sunny windowsill, water it regularly, and you now have a lovely plant.

In 20 years, it may even produce an avocado.

Fresh Tomato Salsa

Sure, you can buy salsa by the vat in any grocery store, but it's not like this stuff. Fresh salsa is something else altogether. Try it.

1 lb.	500 g	perfectly ripe plum tomatoes
½		medium red onion, finely chopped
2		cloves garlic, minced
1 or 2		fresh jalapeño peppers, seeded and minced (or more—hey!)
¼ cup	50 mL	chopped cilantro
2 tbsp.	30 mL	fresh lime juice
1 tsp.	5 mL	salt

Cut the tomatoes in half, crosswise, and gently squeeze out as much of the juicy, seedy pulp as you can. Chop the tomatoes finely (don't liquefy them!) and place them in a bowl. Add the rest of the ingredients, and taste to adjust the seasoning—this is not a scientific formula. You can add and subtract to your heart's content.

Let the salsa sit, at room temperature, for at least 30 minutes before serving.

Is that great, or what?

Makes about 3 cups (750 mL).

Speedy breakfast burrito

Yikes! You're late! But you're hungry. Quick! Make this and run.

Scramble an egg or two or make some scrambled tofu (page 85) and scoop it onto a flour tortilla. (If you have an extra 20 seconds, zap the tortilla in the microwave first.) Slop on a couple of spoonfuls of tomato salsa, sprinkle with some shredded cheese, fold up the bottom, roll in the sides, and eat.

Now get out of here!

Spicy Black Bean Dip

This is one of the fastest dips around—both coming and going. It takes about three minutes to make, and only a little longer to disappear.

1		(19-oz./540 mL) can black beans, drained (2 cups/500 mL home-cooked)
1		clove garlic, squished
½ cup	125 mL	salsa (hot, medium or mild)
2 tbsp.	30 mL	chopped cilantro (optional)
		sour cream and shredded cheese for garnish

Dump the beans, garlic, salsa and cilantro into the container of a blender or food processor and blend until mashed, but not totally smooth. Or, for more texture (and less stuff to clean up), mash the beans in a bowl with a potato masher or a fork, then stir in the salsa, garlic and chopped cilantro.

Scoop into a bowl, top with a dollop of sour cream, and sprinkle with a bit of shredded cheese (and some more cilantro, if you have it). Serve with tortilla chips or vegetable dippers.

Makes about 2½ cups (625 mL).

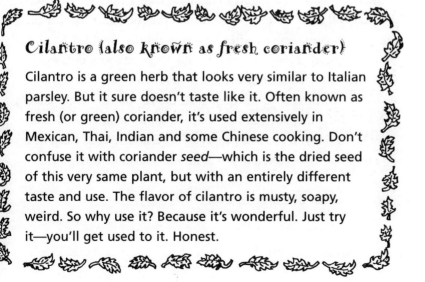

Cilantro (also known as fresh coriander)

Cilantro is a green herb that looks very similar to Italian parsley. But it sure doesn't taste like it. Often known as fresh (or green) coriander, it's used extensively in Mexican, Thai, Indian and some Chinese cooking. Don't confuse it with coriander *seed*—which is the dried seed of this very same plant, but with an entirely different taste and use. The flavor of cilantro is musty, soapy, weird. So why use it? Because it's wonderful. Just try it—you'll get used to it. Honest.

Tzatziki

The secret to great tzatziki is to drain the excess liquid out of both the yogurt and the cucumbers. This will give you a thick, delicious dip that is fresher tasting than anything you can buy ready-made.

3 cups	750 mL	plain yogurt (low-fat is fine)
2		medium cucumbers
1 tsp.	5 mL	salt
1		clove garlic, squished
1 tbsp.	15 mL	olive oil
1 tbsp.	15 mL	chopped fresh mint, dill or chives
		salt and pepper

First, drain the excess liquid from the yogurt. The easiest way to do this is to take a paper coffee filter, place it into a filter holder balanced over a bowl or measuring cup, and dump the yogurt into the filter to drain. If you don't have such equipment, simply dump the yogurt into a strainer lined with a clean dish towel and place it over a bowl to catch the drippings. Either way, let the yogurt drain, refrigerated, for at least 2 hours or overnight.

Meanwhile, peel the cucumbers and grate them on the coarse holes of a grater (or with the shredding blade of a food processor). Place shredded cucumbers in a bowl, add 1 tsp. (5 mL) salt, and let it sit while you wait for the yogurt to drain (at least 1 hour for the cukes). The salt will draw the excess liquid from the cucumbers so that the dip won't become watery. After 1 hour, drain the shredded cucumber thoroughly and, if you want to be really fanatical about this, squeeze the remaining water out by hand. Plunk into a bowl.

Finally, dump the thickened yogurt into the bowl with the cucumber, add the garlic, olive oil and chopped mint (or whatever you're using). Season with salt and pepper to taste, and serve as a dip with pita bread or fresh vegetables, or as an accompaniment to grilled vegetables.

Makes about 2½ cups (625 mL).

Baba Ghanouj

Adjust the amount of garlic to suit your taste—this makes a medium-garlicky dip. You can even use roasted garlic (see next page) if you prefer a mellower garlic flavor.

1		medium eggplant
¼ cup	50 mL	tahini (page 22)
¼ cup	50 mL	lemon juice
2		cloves garlic, squished
		salt to taste
		olive oil (optional)

Prick the eggplant all over with a fork (this is necessary to avoid it exploding) and bake at 450° F (230° C) for about 1 hour, until blackened and soft. Or, place the eggplant on a foil pan in a covered barbecue and cook over medium heat, turning once or twice, until charred and soft. The barbecue method will produce a smokier taste. Which, in this case, is a good thing.

Cut a slit down the length of the eggplant, scoop the mushy insides into a bowl and mash with a fork. Add all the rest of the ingredients, mixing well with a fork. This can be done in a food processor, if you prefer, but be careful not to overprocess the mixture—it should have a little texture.

Spoon the baba ghanouj into a bowl and serve with pita bread or vegetable dippers.

Makes about 2 cups (500 mL).

Eggplant

Resist, if you possibly can, buying the hugest eggplant monstrosity at the market. Small to medium-sized eggplants are likely to be less bitter and seedy. A fresh eggplant should be shiny and firm with no bruises or brown spots. The most familiar type is the bulbous purple-black type of eggplant. These are useful when you want meaty slices or chunks or when you want to roast one whole for a dip. But the long, thin, oriental eggplants are wonderful for cutting up in a stir-fry or vegetable stew, or for slicing in half lengthwise for the grill.

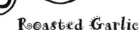

Roasted Garlic

Once you've done a batch of roasted garlic, you'll find a zillion uses for the stuff. You can serve a whole head as an appetizer (really), or squish out the pulp and use it to season salad dressing or mashed potatoes. Roasting turns garlic from a wild and uncivilized maniac into an affable, mellow eccentric. Sort of like when your Uncle Chuckie got married.

4		whole heads of garlic
1 tbsp.	15 mL	olive or vegetable oil
¼ cup	50 mL	vegetable broth or water
¼ tsp.	1 mL	salt

Without breaking up the heads, remove any excess papery skin from the garlic. Keep the heads intact. With a sharp knife, cut a thin slice from the top (pointy end) of each head, just to expose the innards of the cloves slightly. Arrange the garlic heads, cut side up, in a small baking dish, drizzle with the olive or vegetable oil, then pour the vegetable broth or water into the bottom of the dish. Sprinkle lightly with salt, and cover. Bake at 375° F (190° C) for 1 hour, uncovering the dish for the last 10 minutes of baking time.

That's all.

Now, go and have your way with it.

The Best Appetizer in the World

This is it. Here's what you do. For each person, roast one whole head of garlic. Place each roasted garlic on a plate, accompanied by a slice of goat cheese and sliced French bread. To eat—smear goat cheese on the bread, squish out a clove of garlic on top, and eat. Do I lie?

Mexican Meltdown

This wonderfully gloppy cheesy goop will make you instantly famous.
Be prepared to make it for every party.

1 tbsp.	15 mL	olive oil
1		onion, chopped
4		green onions, chopped
2 or 3		jalapeño peppers
½		medium sweet red pepper, chopped
2		medium tomatoes, peeled, seeded and chopped
2		cloves garlic, squished
¼ cup	50 mL	whipping or table cream
4 cups	1 L	shredded Cheddar or Monterey Jack cheese
2 tbsp.	30 mL	all-purpose flour
1 tsp.	5 mL	ground cumin
		salt and pepper to taste

Heat the olive oil in a large skillet over medium heat. Add chopped onion, green onions, chopped jalapeño peppers and red peppers, and cook, stirring, until the onions are soft—6 to 8 minutes. Stir in tomatoes and garlic and let simmer for 5 minutes, until tomatoes begin to soften. Stir in the cream.

Meanwhile, toss the cheese with the flour and cumin, then add to the tomato mixture in the skillet. Season to taste. Cook just long enough to melt the cheese.

Serve warm with tortilla chips for dipping.

Cheese

Use whatever cheese you happen to have. Recipe calls for Cheddar and all you have is Swiss? Use it. The taste will be different but—who knows?— you may even like it better. Rule of thumb: Try to substitute cheeses of the same consistency (soft, medium or hard) for one another.

Veggie Pâté

This stuff looks (and almost tastes) so much like chopped liver that it's uncanny. Serve it with crackers or thinly sliced French bread, and let everyone wonder if you've started eating meat again.

3 tbsp.	45 mL	vegetable oil
2		medium onions, chopped
1		(19-oz./540 mL) can lentils, drained (2 cups/500 mL home-cooked)
4		hard-cooked eggs, peeled and quartered
1 tbsp.	15 mL	peanut butter
½ tsp.	2 mL	salt
		pepper to taste

Heat the oil in a small skillet, add the chopped onions, and cook over medium-low heat until the onions are golden brown—10 to 15 minutes. Remove from heat and set aside.

If you have a food processor, dump the sautéed onions, the lentils, and the hard-cooked eggs into the container and process until finely chopped, but not totally smooth. Add the peanut butter, salt and pepper. Process until blended. If you don't have a food processor, chop the ingredients as finely as possible, then, with a fork or potato masher, mash everything together in a bowl until almost (but not quite) smooth.

Chill before serving.

Makes about 3 cups (750 mL).

Artichokes—The Porcupine of the Vegetable World

For a fun appetizer, buy one fresh artichoke per person. Trim the prickly bits, the stem and any discolored leaves. Steam for 30 minutes, or until a leaf can be removed easily. Serve hot with Pseudo-Hollandaise Sauce (page 111) for dipping, or cold with Vinaigrette Dressing (page 77).

To eat, pull off the leaves one at a time. Dip the leaf base into the dipping sauce and scrape it between your teeth to remove the fleshy part. Discard the fibrous leaf. Continue until you get to the fuzzy middle or "choke". Remove, and eat the delicious bottom part.

There. Don't you feel sophisticated?

Salsa Cheese Bites

This great munchie can be thrown together in minutes, with stuff you probably already have around the house. If you like your food really zingy, use chopped fresh jalapeño peppers instead of the canned chilies.

2 cups	500 mL	shredded Cheddar cheese
2 cups	500 mL	shredded Monterey Jack cheese
2		(4.5-oz./127 mL) cans chopped green chilies
1 cup	250 mL	biscuit mix—homemade (page 192) or a commercial brand
4		eggs, beaten
½ cup	125 mL	milk
½ cup	125 mL	salsa

Sprinkle the cheeses evenly over the bottom of a greased 9 x 13 inch (22 x 33 cm) baking pan. Spread the chilies over the cheeses.

In a mixing bowl, beat together the biscuit mix, eggs and milk. Pour this mixture over the cheese and chilies, spreading it out to cover as much as possible. Dollop the salsa over top of everything. Bake at 425° F (220° C) for 25 to 30 minutes, until set. Let cool for about 10 minutes before cutting into squares. Serve warm.

Makes about 25 squares.

Zucchini Appetizers

Some people will flee at the mere mention of the word zucchini. This is unfortunate, since it really has some wonderful uses. This, for instance.

3 cups	750 mL	shredded zucchini
1 cup	250 mL	biscuit mix—homemade (see page 192 or a commercial brand
½ cup	125 mL	grated Parmesan cheese
1		small onion, finely chopped
2 tbsp.	30 mL	chopped fresh parsley
2 tbsp.	30 mL	chopped fresh basil (or 2 tsp./10 mL dried)
½ tsp.	2 mL	hot pepper sauce (if you like that sort of thing)
1 tsp.	5 mL	salt
¼ tsp.	1 mL	pepper
⅓ cup	75 mL	vegetable oil
4		eggs, beaten

In a large bowl, combine all the ingredients, mixing well. Spread into a well-greased 9 x 13-inch (22 x 33 cm) baking dish. Bake at 350° F (180° C) for 25 to 30 minutes, until just beginning to brown lightly on top.

Cut into squares or diamonds or triangles or trapezoids and serve hot or at room temperature.

Makes at least 24 squares. Let your guests just *try* to guess what's in it.

Quesadillas

Is it an appetizer? Is it a main dish? Who cares? It's fast, good and fun.

You'll definitely need:
Flour tortillas—any size
Salsa
Shredded Monterey Jack or Cheddar cheese

You may also want to add:
Refried beans—homemade (page 36) or canned
Chopped jalapeño peppers
Chopped onions, sweet peppers, olives, tomatoes, whatever

Start with one flour tortilla. Spread it—to within ½ inch (1 cm) of the edge—with refried beans, if you're using them. Spoon the salsa over the beans, then sprinkle with shredded cheese and whatever else you're using. Slap a second tortilla on top, pressing down to squash the two together like a sandwich.

Now heat a large frying pan or griddle—no oil or anything—over medium heat for a minute or two. Place the quesadilla on the pan and cook, squishing down lightly with a spatula, until the bottom begins to brown slightly. Flip the quesadilla over to allow the other side to brown slightly, and the cheese inside to melt. Remove to a cutting board and cut into wedges with a pizza cutter or a sharp knife.

Repeat until you are full.

Homemade Refried Beans

Make a double batch of these refried beans and keep them in the freezer to use in quesadillas or wherever you want to put them.

1 tbsp.	15 mL	vegetable oil
1		onion, chopped
1		clove garlic, squished
2		(19-oz./540 mL) cans pinto, kidney or Mexican pink beans (4 cups/1 L home-cooked)
		salt and pepper to taste

In a very large, heavy skillet, heat the vegetable oil over medium heat. Add the chopped onion and garlic and cook, stirring, until the onion is quite soft—about 10 minutes. Drain the canned beans (if you're using canned), reserving the liquid. Now dump in the beans and cook, mashing them with a potato masher or a wooden spoon, and stirring almost constantly. Add a bit of the bean cooking water or the liquid from the cans to the beans and continue cooking, stirring and mashing, until the mixture is thick and the beans are about half mashed. Season to taste.

Serve sprinkled with cheese as a side dish with rice or tortillas, as a filling for burritos or as an ingredient in quesadillas or nachos.

Makes about 3 cups (750 mL).

Muncho Grande Platter

You cannot resist.

1		(19-oz./540 mL) can black or pinto beans (2 cups/500 mL home-cooked)
½ cup	125 mL	chopped or sliced black olives
¼ cup	50 mL	chopped onion
1		clove garlic, squished
2 tbsp.	30 mL	lime juice
1 tbsp.	15 mL	olive or vegetable oil
½ tsp.	2 mL	ground cumin
¼ tsp.	1 mL	hot pepper flakes
1 cup	250 mL	spreadable cream cheese (8-oz./ 250 mL pkg)
1		green or red sweet pepper, chopped
2		green onions, chopped
½ cup	125 mL	shredded Monterey Jack or Cheddar cheese

In a bowl, combine the beans, olives, chopped onion, garlic, lime juice, oil, cumin and hot pepper flakes. Stir, then cover and refrigerate for 1 or 2 hours, to allow the flavors to blend.

Just before serving, spread the cream cheese out on a serving plate. Spoon the bean mixture over the top, then sprinkle with chopped sweet pepper, green onions and shredded cheese.

Serve with tortilla chips for dipping.

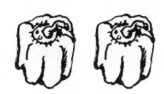

3. Soups From Scratch

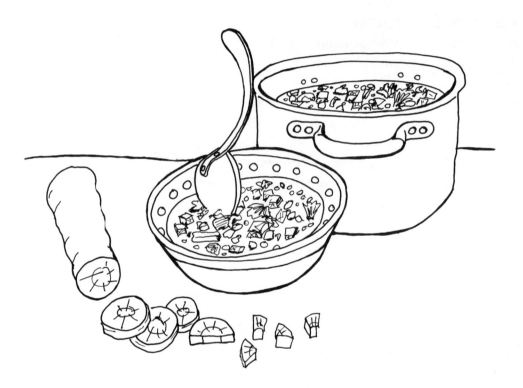

Vegetable Broth

The following vegetable broth recipe (and the roasted veggie variation) can be used whenever you need a good, basic vegetable stock. Cook up a big batch and freeze it in small (2 cup/500 mL) containers so you'll always have some homemade broth to use when you need it.

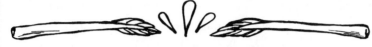

Golden Vegetable Broth

This cheerful golden broth is close enough to chicken broth to make it a good substitute in any recipe that calls for such a thing. It's a great all-purpose vegetable broth.

4		medium carrots, cut into chunks
2		medium onions, cut into chunks
2		parsnips, cut into chunks
1		leek, carefully washed and sliced
1		head garlic, separated into cloves, but not peeled
1 cup	250 mL	coarsely chopped fresh parsley
12 cups	3 L	water
1 tbsp.	15 mL	salt
1 tsp.	5 mL	turmeric (*aha!* the secret!)
¼ tsp.	1 mL	pepper (or more, to taste)

Combine all the ingredients in a large stock pot and bring to a boil over high heat. Cover the pot, lower the heat and simmer for 1½ to 2 hours.

Let the soup cool, then strain the soggy vegetables out and have your way with the broth. The soup vegetables, alas, are history.

Makes about 10 cups (2.5 L).

Roasted Veggie Variation

For a darker broth, closer in flavor to beef than chicken, try this:

Toss the carrots, onions, parsnips, leek and garlic with 1 tbsp. (15 mL) of olive oil. Place in a large roasting pan and bake at 400° F (200° C), stirring a few times, until the vegetables are beginning to brown—about 45 minutes. Remove the pan from the oven, pour in 2 cups (500 mL) of water and stir around to dissolve the brown bits from the bottom of the pan. Dump everything into a stock pot and continue the recipe as in Golden Vegetable Broth.

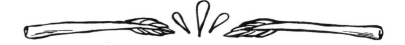

The Stock Bag

Instead of throwing out all those vegetable trimmings (peels, tips, leaves, all the junk you don't exactly want to eat), stuff them into a bag and toss it into the freezer. You can add to the bag whenever you have something to throw in, and use it when you're ready to make a pot of stock. It looks disgusting, but you'll be boiling everything, so it certainly can't kill you.

Try:
- Potato peels (*not* the eyes or any green parts)
- Pea pods
- Onion ends (the green parts too!)
- The insides of a green pepper
- Celery leaves
- Carrot peels
- Mushroom stems
- Wilted beans
- Mushy tomatoes

Split Pea Soup

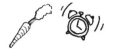

You'd think that something like split pea soup would take hours to make, wouldn't you? It doesn't.

2 cups	500 mL	split peas (green or yellow—it doesn't matter)
8 cups	2 L	cold water
2		stalks celery, chopped
2		medium carrots, chopped
2		small onions, chopped
1 tsp.	5 mL	salt
½ tsp.	2 mL	pepper
2 tbsp.	15 mL	chopped fresh parsley

Rinse the split peas in several changes of water, then place them in a large saucepan or Dutch oven. Add the cold water and bring to a boil over medium-high heat. Lower the heat to a simmer and cook, covered, for about 20 minutes, stirring occasionally, until the peas are soft.

Add the celery, carrots, onions, salt, pepper and parsley. Bring back to a boil, and simmer, covered, for another 30 minutes, until the vegetables are tender and the split peas have almost completely disintegrated. Taste and adjust seasoning, if necessary.

Makes 6 to 8 servings.

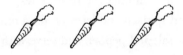

Chick-Pea and Tomato Soup

A big bowl (or two) of this soup, a loaf of good bread and it's dinner. Well, okay, maybe just a sliver of apple pie and a small scoop of ice cream too …

Vegetable Broth

In any recipe that calls for vegetable broth, you can use homemade (page 39), canned or vegetable broth made from a good quality bouillon cube or powder. Keep in mind, however, that canned and powdered broths tend to be saltier than homemade, so taste before adding salt to the recipe

2 tbsp.	30 mL	olive or vegetable oil
1		large onion, chopped
2		medium zucchini, cut into ¼ inch (.5 cm) cubes
2		cloves garlic, squished
1		(28-oz./796 mL) can diced tomatoes
1 tbsp.	15 mL	tomato paste
4 cups	1 L	vegetable broth
1		(19-oz./540 mL) can chick-peas, drained (2 cups/500 mL home-cooked)
10-oz.	284 g	package spinach, washed and coarsely chopped
2 tsp.	10 mL	salt
¼ tsp.	1 mL	pepper
		grated Parmesan cheese for sprinkling

Heat the oil in a large saucepan or Dutch oven. Add the chopped onion, zucchini and garlic, and cook, stirring, for 6 to 8 minutes over medium heat, until the vegetables are just softened. Pour in the tomatoes, tomato paste, vegetable broth and chick-peas. Bring to a boil, then lower the heat and simmer for 10 minutes.

Add the shredded spinach and let cook for a minute or two, until wilted. Season with salt and pepper, and serve with Parmesan cheese to sprinkle at the table.

Makes 6 to 8 servings.

Quick Lentil Soup

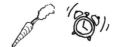

A substantial soup in less than half an hour. You need this recipe.

1 tbsp.	15 mL	olive or vegetable oil
1		onion, chopped
2		cloves garlic, squished
1		medium carrot, chopped
1		stalk celery, chopped
1 tsp.	5 mL	ground cumin
1		(28-oz./796 mL) can diced tomatoes
1		(19-oz./540 mL) can lentils, drained
		(2 cups/500 mL home-cooked)
1½ cups	375 mL	vegetable broth
1 tsp.	5 mL	salt

Heat the oil in a large saucepan or Dutch oven and cook the chopped onion, garlic, carrot, celery and cumin over medium heat, stirring once in a while, for about 10 minutes.

Add the diced tomatoes and all their juice, the lentils, the vegetable broth and the salt, and bring to a boil over medium-high heat. Lower the heat and let the soup simmer for about 15 minutes, or until the vegetables are tender. Adjust seasoning and serve.

Done.

Makes 4 servings.

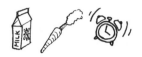

Creamy Carrot Soup

This soup makes you feel healthy just by looking at it. And eating it is even better.

1 tbsp.	30 mL	butter or vegetable oil
1		small onion, chopped
1 lb.	500 g	carrots, diced (about 6 medium carrots)
2 cups	500 mL	vegetable broth
2 tbsp.	30 mL	raw white rice
1 tsp.	5 mL	salt
		pepper to taste
½ tsp.	2 mL	crumbled dried thyme
1		bay leaf
1½ cups	375 mL	milk (or soy milk)
1 tbsp.	15 mL	chopped chives (for garnish)

In a medium saucepan, heat the butter or vegetable oil over medium heat. Add the chopped onion and cook, stirring, until softened—about 5 minutes. Add the carrots, broth, rice, salt, pepper, thyme and bay leaf. Cover and bring to a boil. Reduce the heat and let simmer for about 20 minutes or until carrots and rice are tender. Fish out the bay leaf and discard.

With a slotted spoon, transfer the carrots and rice to the container of a blender or food processor, leaving as much of the cooking liquid behind as you can. Purée the mixture. Then, with the machine still running, pour the cooking liquid in through the feed tube or hole in the lid of the container. Blend until the soup is very smooth. Pour the blended soup back into the saucepan and bring to a boil, stirring. Add the milk and heat through without boiling.

Serve soup sprinkled with chopped chives.

Makes 4 servings.

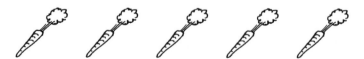

Old-Fashioned Potato Soup

Here's a wonderfully comforting soup that takes about half an hour to make. Perfect for a gloomy fall day when everything seems to be going wrong. Serve this with Tomato Garlic Green Beans (page 180) and Sweet and Sour Roasted Beet Salad (page 59) for a Moscow-inspired supper.

2 tbsp.	30 mL	butter or vegetable oil
2		medium potatoes, peeled and diced
2		medium onions, chopped
2		stalks celery, chopped
2		cloves garlic, squished
1½ cups	375 mL	vegetable broth
1½ cups	375 mL	milk (or soy milk)
		salt and pepper to taste
		chopped chives or paprika for garnish

Melt the butter in a large saucepan or Dutch oven over medium heat. Add the potatoes, onions, celery and garlic and cook, stirring, for 6 to 8 minutes, until the onions are just beginning to soften. Add the vegetable broth, bring to a boil, then cover and simmer for 20 to 25 minutes, until the potatoes are completely falling-apart tender. Let cool for just a few minutes.

With a potato masher (or a fork), mash the soup in the pot until there are no big lumps left. Pour about half of the mashed soup into the container of a blender or food processor. Add the milk and blend until completely smooth. Return the blended mixture to the mashed mixture in the saucepan, and stir to combine. This will give you a semi-smooth soup, with just enough texture to give you something to chew on. If you want a completely smooth soup, blend the whole business in the blender (you may have to do it in two batches).

Adjust the seasoning with salt and pepper, and heat through but don't boil. Sprinkle each serving with chopped chives or a dusting of paprika.

Makes 4 to 5 servings.

Cream of Cauliflower Soup

It seems almost, well, disrespectful to throw something as beautiful as a cauliflower into the blender. Well, you'll get over it.

1		small cauliflower (whole, raw, completely intact!)
1		small carrot, sliced
3 cups	750 mL	vegetable broth
1/3 cup	75 mL	raw white rice
2 cups	500 mL	milk (or soy milk)
1 tbsp.	15 mL	lemon juice
1/2 tsp.	2 mL	salt
1/4 tsp.	1 mL	cayenne
1/4 tsp.	1 mL	nutmeg
		sour cream or yogurt (optional, for garnish)

Trim the leaves from your whole, raw, completely intact cauliflower and plunk it into a big pot of boiling water. Cook for 3 minutes, then drain and let cool until you can handle it. Cut into pieces— this doesn't have to be a big process, you'll be blending it up later anyway. Dump the cauliflower into a large saucepan. Discard the cooking water.

Add the sliced carrot, the vegetable broth and the rice. Bring to a boil over medium-high heat, then lower the heat, and simmer, stirring once in a while, for about 30 minutes. The rice should be completely cooked. Remove from heat and stir in the milk.

Place the soup in the container of a blender or food processor and blend until completely smooth. You'll probably have to do this in two or three batches—it's quite a lot. Return the blended soup to the saucepan, add the lemon juice, salt, cayenne and nutmeg, and heat until warmed through.

Serve hot or cold—with a dollop of sour cream or yogurt in each bowl.

Makes 6 servings.

Mushroom Barley Soup

It's a dark and stormy night. But inside the kitchen you're warm and cozy because you're about to have a delicious bowl of this very comfy soup. Serve this with Oven-Roasted Carrot and Sweet Potato Casserole (page 147) and Bulgur Pilaf (page 174).

3 tbsp.	45 mL	butter (or vegetable oil)
2		small onions, chopped
2		medium carrots, chopped
1		stalk celery, chopped
2		cloves garlic, squished
1 lb.	500 g	mushrooms, sliced
3 quarts	3 L	vegetable broth
1 cup	250 mL	barley
1 tsp.	5 mL	crumbled dried thyme
2 tbsp.	30 mL	chopped fresh parsley
2 tbsp.	30 mL	chopped fresh dill weed
		salt and pepper to taste

In a large pot or Dutch oven, melt the butter over medium heat. Add the onions, carrots, celery and garlic and cook, stirring, for about 10 minutes or until tender. Add the sliced mushrooms and let cook for another 5 to 8 minutes, until the mushrooms have let out their juices, and the liquid is beginning to evaporate.

Now add the vegetable broth, barley and thyme, and bring to a boil. Cover the pot with a lid, lower the heat to a simmer, and let the soup cook, stirring occasionally, for 1½ hours. If it is becoming too thick, add more water. Add the chopped parsley and dill, simmer for another 15 minutes, and season with salt and pepper to taste.

Makes 8 to 10 servings.

Phenomenal Minestrone Soup

If you buy your Parmesan cheese as a chunk, save the rinds (in the freezer, if necessary) to toss into this soup. You won't believe the difference it makes in the flavor. Really. This is amazing accompanied by Fabulous Focaccia (page 190) and Peach and Banana Flambé (page 206).

2 tbsp.	30 mL	olive or vegetable oil
2		medium onions, chopped
4		cloves garlic, squished
4 cups	1 L	water
2		medium carrots, sliced
2		stalks celery, sliced
1		(28-oz./796 mL) can tomatoes, broken up
3		3-inch (8 cm) pieces Parmesan cheese rind (optional)
1 tsp.	5 mL	salt
¼ tsp.	2 mL	pepper
1 cup	250 mL	green beans, cut into 1-inch (2.5 cm) pieces
½ cup	125 mL	smallish macaroni (uncooked)—like elbows or shells
1		medium zucchini, sliced
3 cups	750 mL	shredded raw spinach (about half of a 10-oz./284 g bag)
1		(19-oz./540 mL) can white or red kidney beans (2 cups/500 mL home-cooked)

Heat the oil in a large stock pot or Dutch oven. Add the onion and garlic, and cook over medium heat, stirring occasionally, for about 5 minutes, until the onion begins to soften. Add the water, carrots, celery, tomatoes, cheese rinds, salt and pepper. Bring to a boil over medium-high heat, then reduce the heat to low. Cover and simmer for 30 to 40 minutes.

Add the green beans and macaroni and let cook for 10 minutes. Add the zucchini, spinach and beans and cook for another 10 to 15 minutes.

Fish out and remove the cheese rinds and serve with additional grated Parmesan cheese to sprinkle on top.

Makes 6 to 8 servings.

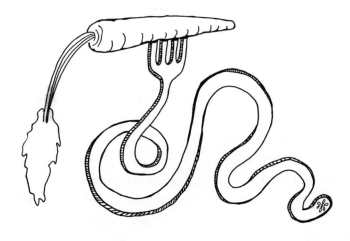

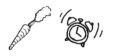

Curried Red Lentil Soup

Little red lentils are a great thing to keep around—they cook really quickly, and don't require any long soaking. This soup is thick enough to be spooned over cooked rice as a main dish, or even rolled into chapatis or tortillas.

1¼ cups	300 mL	red lentils
½ cup	125 mL	raw white rice
¼ cup	50 mL	olive or vegetable oil
1		medium onion, chopped
2 tbsp.	30 mL	curry powder
6 cups	1.5 L	vegetable broth
½ tsp.	2 mL	salt
		yogurt or lemon wedges (optional)

Measure the lentils and the rice into a medium bowl, and rinse in several changes of water, draining off the cloudy water and repeating until the water remains clear. Cover with fresh warm water and let soak for a few minutes.

While the lentils and rice are soaking, heat the oil in a large saucepan over medium heat. Add the onion, and let cook until softened—about 5 minutes. Add the curry powder and cook, stirring, for 2 minutes. Pour in the vegetable broth, and bring the mixture to a boil. Meanwhile, drain the lentils and rice, and dump into the saucepan. As soon as the soup begins to boil, reduce the heat, cover the pot and let simmer, stirring occasionally, until the lentils and rice are tender—about 20 minutes.

Now, you can serve the soup as it is, and it's quite fine. Or, you can blend the whole business in a blender or food processor for a smooth and creamy lentil soup. Or (best of both worlds) blend about half the soup, and stir the blended and unblended parts together for a semi-smooth result. It will still be quite thick—you can add a little more broth to thin it, if you like. Add the salt (some canned vegetable broths are already quite salty, so taste it first), heat through and serve with a dollop of yogurt or a wedge of lemon.

Makes about 4 servings.

Black Bean Soup

This classic soup is a full meal in itself. Keep a bottle of hot pepper sauce on stand-by at the table if you like your soup a little spicy.

2 cups	500 mL	dry black beans
1 tbsp.	15 mL	vegetable oil
1		onion, chopped
4		cloves garlic, squished
1		stalk celery, chopped
10 cups	2.5 L	water or vegetable broth
1		bay leaf
		pinch each summer savory, thyme, sage (or whatever)
		salt and pepper to taste
2 tbsp.	30 mL	lime or lemon juice (or more, to taste)
		yogurt or sour cream for garnish

Rinse beans thoroughly and place in a large pot with plenty of water to cover at least 2 inches (5 cm) over the beans. Soak using either the long soak or quick soak method (page 53). Drain and rinse.

Heat oil in a large pot or Dutch oven over medium heat. Sauté onion, 2 of the squished garlic cloves and celery for 6 to 8 minutes, until onion is tender. Add the soaked, drained beans to the pot, along with water or broth, bay leaf, savory, thyme and sage. Bring to a boil over high heat, then reduce heat, cover, and let simmer for 1½ hours. Add the remaining 2 squished garlic cloves and continue to cook for another 1 to 1½ hours, until the beans are soft. If the soup is very thick, you can add some water to thin it.

Fish the bay leaf out of the soup and dump about half of the soup into a blender or food processor. Purée, then return the puréed mixture to the pot with the rest of the soup. Stir in salt and pepper to taste and lime or lemon juice. Heat through, and serve with a garnish of yogurt or sour cream, if you like.

Makes 6 to 8 servings.

Hot Summer Day Variation

Make this delicious Black Bean Soup soup and chill it. Just before serving, stir in some buttermilk, and serve with a dollop of yogurt and some chopped avocado.

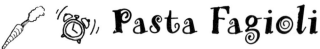

Pasta Fagioli

A cross between a soup and a pasta. Let's not nitpick. Whatever it is, it's good. This is perfect accompanied by Parmesan Onion Bread (page 194).

2 tbsp.	30 mL	olive or vegetable oil
1		carrot, chopped
1		stalk celery, chopped
1		onion, chopped
2		garlic cloves, chopped
6 cups	1.5 L	vegetable broth
1		(19-oz./540 mL) can white kidney beans, undrained and totally mashed with a fork (2 cups/500 mL home-cooked)
1		(19-oz./540 mL) can red kidney beans, drained (2 cups/500 mL home-cooked)
1 cup	250 mL	small pasta—like very small shells or ditali (little tubes)
		salt and black pepper to taste

Heat the olive or vegetable oil in a large saucepan or Dutch oven. Cook the carrot, celery, onion and garlic over medium heat, stirring occasionally, for 7 to 10 minutes, or until the onions are lightly browned.

Add the vegetable broth, mashed white kidney beans and unmashed red kidney beans. Bring to a boil over high heat. Add the pasta, and cook for 8 to 10 minutes, until the pasta is cooked but not mushy (taste one to see). Season with salt and black pepper to taste.

Makes about 6 servings.

Cooking Dried Beans—the Essential Guide

Of course you can use canned beans. Most of the time, even. But inevitably you will have to learn how to cook dried beans. It's simply your destiny. So you may as well learn now.

All dried beans need to be soaked in water before cooking. This allows the beans to become partially rehydrated so that they will cook more evenly. There are two ways to do this—the long soak method, and the quick soak method. Either method will give you good results. First rinse your beans thoroughly, and pick them over to remove any alien bits and stones that may have gotten mixed in. Place the beans in a large pot or Dutch oven and add enough water to cover the beans by at least 2 inches (5 cm).

For the **long soak method**, simply let the beans soak for at least 12 hours or overnight at room temperature (or in the refrigerator). Drain, discarding the soaking water, then rinse and proceed with your recipe.

For the **quick soak method**, bring the beans and water to a boil over high heat. Let cook for 5 minutes, then cover the pot and turn off the burner. Let the beans soak for 1 hour at room temperature. Drain, discarding the soaking water, rinse and proceed with your recipe.

To cook your soaked beans, add enough water to the soaked beans to come at least 1 inch (2.5 cm) above the level of the beans in the pot. Add a peeled whole onion, a couple of whole garlic cloves, maybe a slice of ginger, and bring to a boil over medium heat. *Do not add salt* (this will toughen the skins and prevent them from cooking properly). Lower the heat to a simmer, cover the pot and let the beans cook until they are soft. Depending on the type of bean and the freshness, this can take anywhere from 30 minutes to 2 hours. Just keep testing the beans every 15 minutes or so until they are tender.

Now that wasn't so hard, was it?

African Peanut Soup

If you think that peanut butter should only ever be seen in a sandwich, think again. The peanut is a legume, and probably has more in common with a kidney bean than it does with a walnut or an almond. If you need more convincing, try this soup.

1 tbsp.	15 mL	vegetable oil
2		onions, chopped
2		carrots, chopped
4 cups	1 L	vegetable broth
¼ cup	50 mL	raw white rice
½ cup	125 mL	smooth peanut butter
½ tsp.	2 mL	hot pepper sauce
		salt to taste

Heat the oil in a large saucepan over medium heat. Add the onions and carrots and cook, stirring, until the onions are soft—8 to 10 minutes. Add the vegetable broth and bring to a boil. Cover the pot, then lower the heat to a simmer and cook for 20 minutes.

Dump the soup into a blender and blend until smooth. Pour the soup back into the pot, add the rice, and cook, covered, for 15 minutes, until the rice is soft. Stir in the peanut butter, the hot pepper sauce and salt to taste. Heat through and serve.

Makes 4 servings.

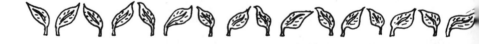

Cold Zucchini Soup

Think of this, if you must, as a salad. A very sloppy salad. It is absolutely delicious, almost ridiculously easy to make and the most refreshing way to start a summer meal.

4		smallish zucchinis
2 cups	500 mL	water
2 tbsp.	30 mL	chopped fresh dill weed
1 tsp.	5 mL	salt
1 cup	250 mL	sour cream (regular or low fat)

Wash the zucchinis and trim off the ends. Shred zukes using the coarse holes of a grater or with the shredding blade of a food processor.

Dump the zucchini shreds into a medium saucepan. Add the water, the dill weed and the salt. Bring to a boil, then lower the heat and let simmer for 10 minutes. Remove from heat, cool, then chill for several hours or overnight.

Just before you're ready to eat, measure the sour cream into a small bowl. Stir in a few spoonfuls of the soup to thin it, then stir the sour cream mixture back into the soup, mixing until it's all creamy.

Ladle the soup into bowls, and garnish each serving with a floating island of sour cream and, perhaps, a sprig of fresh dill.

Makes 4 to 6 servings.

4. Serious Salads and Dynamic Dressings

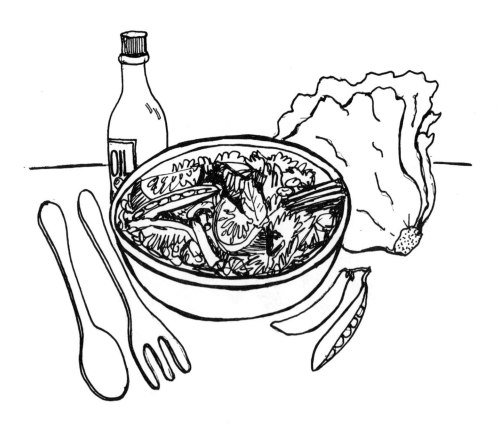

Serious Salads

Fancy French Potato Salad

Magnifique.

6		large new potatoes (or about 3 lbs./ 2.5 kg small ones)
¼ cup	50 mL	olive oil
¼ cup	50 mL	vegetable broth
¼ cup	50 mL	white wine (or use more vegetable broth)
2 tbsp.	30 mL	Dijon mustard
2 tbsp.	30 mL	cider or white wine vinegar
2 tbsp.	30 mL	capers (optional, but fancy and delicious)
4		green onions, chopped
		salt and pepper to taste

Steam or boil the potatoes, without peeling them, until they are tender when poked with the point of a sharp knife. Drain and return to the pot, letting any excess water evaporate.

While the potatoes are boiling, whisk together the olive oil, vegetable broth, wine, mustard, vinegar, capers and chopped green onions to make the dressing.

Cut the potatoes into fairly thick slices while still warm, then toss the warm potatoes gently with the dressing—be careful not to mush up the slices. Let stand for at least 1 hour before serving. Toss again just before serving.

Makes 4 to 6 servings.

> **Mustard**
>
> You can't go wrong if you keep a jar of Dijon mustard around the house. The regular yellow hot dog type of mustard is too harsh to use for most salad dressings or cooking purposes.

Citrus Spinach Salad

Use the freshest, crispest spinach you can find to make this salad. For a chic, but not obnoxious meal, serve this with Roasted Tomato Fettuccine (page 98), Fabulous Focaccia (page 190) and Truly Astonishing Tofu Chocolate Mousse (page 207).

6 cups	**1.5 L**	**fresh spinach, washed, dried and torn into pieces**
1		**orange, peeled and cut into chunks**
½		**small sweet onion (Spanish or Vidalia are good), thinly sliced**

In a large bowl, toss together the spinach, the orange chunks and the sliced onion. Serve with a basic vinaigrette dressing (page 77) sweetened with just a pinch or two of sugar.

Gorgeous.

Makes 3 or 4 servings.

A Simple Green Salad

Begin with lettuce. Try several kinds—mix them up.

Add some other greens: escarole, endive, radicchio, arugula. Be brave. Experiment.

Wash and dry everything well—use a salad spinner if you have one.

Now add stuff. Tomato chunks, cucumber slices, carrot shreds, red pepper, red onion, red cabbage, radishes. Whatever. Or don't add anything.

Drizzle with just enough dressing to lightly coat the leaves, toss gently and serve immediately.

There. Simple, isn't it?

Sweet and Sour Roasted Beet Salad

Remember those yucky gluey beets with the sweet sauce you always hated? Well, this is not them. Totally.

1 lb.	500 g	fresh beets, peeled and cut into chunks (5 or 6 medium beets)
1		medium Spanish onion, thinly sliced
¼ cup	50 mL	olive oil
2 tbsp.	30 mL	balsamic vinegar
2 tbsp.	30 mL	water
2		cloves garlic, chopped
1 tbsp.	15 mL	chopped fresh mint leaves
1 tsp.	5 mL	salt
¼ tsp.	1 mL	pepper

Combine all the ingredients in a casserole dish, tossing to mix well. Cover and bake at 350° F (180° C) for 1½ hours, or until the beets are tender.

Chill before serving.

Makes 4 servings.

Balsamic Vinegar

Here's an ingredient which most people hadn't heard of five years ago, and now you run into it everywhere. And for good reason. It's a wonderful seasoning—a little sweet, a little sour. Very nice. Start with a small bottle of the cheapest kind you can get, then work your way up to the good stuff.

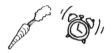

Crunchy Coleslaw

If anything, this salad actually improves with age. Make it the day before you want to serve it to let the dressing have its way with the cabbage.

½		a small head of cabbage, finely shredded (about 6 cups/1.5 L)
1		carrot, grated
1		green pepper, chopped
2		green onions, chopped
¼ cup	50 mL	vegetable oil
2 tbsp.	30 mL	vinegar
½ tsp.	2 mL	salt
¼ tsp.	1 mL	pepper
½ tsp	2 mL	sugar
1 tsp.	5 mL	celery seed

Combine all the ingredients and toss well to mix. That's all, folks.

Makes 4 to 6 servings.

Vaguely Oriental Variation

Try making the coleslaw with Incredible Oriental Dressing (page 67). Omit the oil, vinegar and seasonings from the recipe above and, instead, toss the salad with Incredible Oriental Dressing for something different.

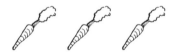

Corn and Tomato Salad

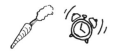

For that extra you-know-what, grill the cooked corn on the barbecue for a few minutes, turning the cobs over so that all sides are lightly charred. Then make the salad. Amazing. This makes a beautiful summer meal accompanied by Crepes filled with Ratatouille (page 92), Barbecued Portobello Burgers (page 161).

4		medium ears of corn, cooked (leftover is fine)
2		medium tomatoes, chopped
½		small red or Spanish onion, chopped
2 tbsp.	30 mL	olive oil
1 tbsp.	15 mL	cider or wine vinegar
¼ cup	50 mL	chopped or shredded fresh basil leaves
		salt and pepper to taste

With a sharp knife, cut the kernels from the ears of corn and dump them into a bowl. Add all the other ingredients, and toss to combine thoroughly.

Serve immediately or let sit for up to an hour at room temperature.

Makes 4 servings.

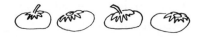

Corn

The minute you pick a cob of corn, the sugars in it that make it taste so good begin their depressing journey toward starch. And who hasn't had the unpleasant surprise of biting into a gorgeous cob of corn only to discover that it tastes like, well, nothing? The moral of this story is that freshness counts—big time—when it comes to buying corn on the cob. If you're buying it at the store, make sure the husks are green and moist, not dried out, and the stringy silk part is damp and fresh looking.

Warm Mushroom Salad

This is such a totally fabulous first course that it will make you famous instantly. It's hardly any work, really, for such a wonderful thing, and is absolutely delicious. Make it with regular white mushrooms, if you like, or with any mixture of fancy-shmancy ones—cremini, shiitake, oyster, portobellos. Serve this with some good French bread, followed by Basic Risotto (page 170) and Fruit Sorbet (page 204).

4 cups	1 L	mixed baby greens (also known as mesclun)
¼ cup	50 mL	olive oil
1		clove garlic, squished
8 oz.	250 g	fresh mushrooms—any kind or combination, sliced
2 tbsp.	30 mL	chopped chives
½ tsp.	2 mL	salt
¼ tsp.	1 mL	pepper
5 oz.	140 g	goat cheese (with or without herbs), cut into 4 pieces
2 tbsp.	30 mL	balsamic vinegar (or cider vinegar with a pinch of sugar)

Divide the mixed baby greens equally among 4 plates. Set aside.

Pour about half of the olive oil into a skillet and heat over medium heat. Add the squished garlic, and cook for a minute or two, just until softened. Dump in the sliced mushrooms and the chopped chives, increase the heat to high, and cook, stirring, for another minute or two. The mushrooms should be just starting to release their liquid. Add salt and pepper, stir, and remove from heat.

With a slotted spoon, remove the mushrooms from the skillet, leaving behind any juices that may have seeped out. Arrange the mushrooms on a baking sheet in 4 piles, and place one piece of goat cheese on top of each pile. Bake at 375° F (190° C) for 5 or 6 minutes, just until the cheese begins to melt. Remove each mushroom/cheese pile from the baking sheet with a spatula, and slide it onto the baby greens on each plate.

Now, quickly, add the rest of the olive oil and the balsamic vinegar to the skillet, place over medium-high heat, and bring to a boil, scraping up any crusty bits from the bottom of the pan. Let cook for a minute or so, then spoon the oil and vinegar dressing evenly over the warm mushrooms and the greens. Serve immediately with some good French bread.

It's just tooooo fabulous.

Makes 4 servings.

Mushrooms

White button mushrooms are the ones you are most familiar with. They're relatively inexpensive and available everywhere, always. But don't stop there. Try portobello mushrooms—gigantic, enormous, huge, walloping mushrooms that can be almost as big as a dinner plate. There are also smaller versions, called cremini mushrooms. And occasionally you can find wild varieties too, like oyster and shiitake mushrooms. Try everything. They won't kill you (usually).

Orange and Red Onion Salad

Serve this to accompany a spicy curry or something wildly Cuban, like Cuban-Style Black Beans (page 139).

4		large seedless oranges
1		small red onion
¼ cup	50 mL	finely chopped cilantro
2 tsp.	10 mL	finely chopped fresh green chili (optional but…)
1 tbsp.	15 mL	vegetable or olive oil
2 tsp.	10 mL	cider or wine vinegar
		salt to taste

Peel the oranges and slice them thinly, crosswise. Place in a bowl. Slice the red onion very thinly into rings, then cut each ring in half, and toss with the orange slices. Add the chopped cilantro, green chili, oil and vinegar. Toss to combine. Season to taste with salt, and serve immediately. Or let stand and serve later.

Makes about 4 servings.

Bean and Barley Salad

The chewy texture of the barley helps this salad hold up when other salads have wilted and gone mushy. It's as good (maybe better) the next day.

1 cup	250 mL	barley
3 cups	750 mL	water
1		(19-oz./540 mL) can red kidney beans, drained (2 cups/500 mL home-cooked)
1		(19-oz./540 mL) can black beans, drained (2 cups/500 mL home-cooked)
1		(14-oz./398 mL) can baby corn cobs, drained and cut into ½-inch (1 cm) pieces
1		green or red pepper, chopped
¼ cup	50 mL	chopped green onion
1		fresh chili pepper, chopped (optional)
¼ cup	50 mL	cider or wine vinegar
½ cup	125 mL	olive oil
1		clove garlic, squished
½ tsp.	2 mL	ground cumin
½ tsp.	2 mL	salt
½ tsp.	2 mL	pepper

In a medium saucepan, combine the barley and the water. Bring to a boil over high heat, then reduce the heat to low, cover and let cook until all the water is absorbed and the barley is tender—35 to 45 minutes. Rinse under cold running water.

In a large bowl, combine the cooked barley, beans, corn, chopped pepper and green onion, and the chopped chili pepper. In a smaller bowl, whisk together the vinegar, oil, garlic, cumin, salt and pepper and add to the bean mixture.

Cover and chill until serving time.

Serves 6 to 8.

Authentic Greek Salad

This salad is wonderful to serve in midsummer, with nice, ripe tomatoes that actually taste like, well, tomatoes. You can make a full meal out of it with the addition of some good bread and a little extra cheese. Or stuff it into a pita pocket for lunch (pack the salad and pita separately, and stuff just before eating). Serve this accompanied by Vegetarian Moussaka (page 144) and Spanakopita (page 148).

4		medium tomatoes, cut into ½-inch (1 cm) chunks
1		long English cucumber, cut into ½-inch (1 cm) chunks
1		red onion, coarsely chopped
¼ cup	50 mL	olive oil
2 tbsp.	30 mL	lemon juice
2 tsp.	10 mL	crumbled dried oregano
½ tsp.	2 mL	salt
¼ tsp.	1 mL	pepper
4 oz.	125 g	feta cheese, crumbled (about 1 cup/ 250 mL)
½ cup	125 mL	brine-cured black olives

In a bowl, toss together the tomatoes, cucumber and red onion.

In a small jar, combine the olive oil, lemon juice, oregano, salt and pepper. Screw on the lid and shake to mix. Pour dressing over the salad, and toss lightly. Just before serving, throw in the feta cheese and olives, and toss again.

Makes 4 to 6 servings.

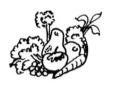

Simple Sesame Noodle Salad

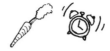

If you happen to have the dressing already made, this (very simple) salad will take you no more than 10 minutes to make—start to finish.

½ lb.	250 g	Japanese soba noodles, spaghettini or vermicelli
1 tsp.	5 mL	Oriental sesame oil
2		green onions, slivered
1		small carrot, grated
½		small onion, coarsely chopped
1		clove garlic
⅓ cup	75 mL	soy sauce
3 tbsp.	45 mL	lemon juice
2 tbsp.	30 mL	water
¼ cup	50 mL	sesame seeds
1½ cups	375 mL	vegetable oil

Boil the noodles or pasta until tender, then drain and rinse under cold running water. Drain very thoroughly and dump into a bowl. Stir in the sesame oil to coat the noodles. Add the slivered green onions and grated carrot. Toss with Incredible Oriental Dressing and sprinkle with additional sesame seeds (toasted, if you have the time) for a little extra crunch.

   Makes 2 to 3 servings.

Incredible Oriental Dressing

Into the container of a blender or food processor, place the onion, garlic, soy sauce, lemon juice, water and sesame seeds. Blend until fairly smooth, then scrape down the sides of the container and replace the lid. With the motor running, pour the oil in through the small opening in the lid, in a thin stream. Blend until smooth and thickened.

   Makes about 2 cups (500 mL).

   (This dressing is really nifty on coleslaw too, try it.)

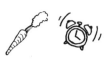

Tofu Egg Salad

Stuffed into a pita, piled onto a fresh bun—this is so good, you'll never miss the egg.

½ lb.	250 g	regular tofu (about 2 medium squares), cut into ¼-inch (.5 cm) dice
¼ tsp.	1 mL	turmeric
1		stalk celery, minced
¼		small onion, minced
¼ cup	50 mL	tofu mayonnaise (see page 82)
1 tsp.	5 mL	Dijon mustard
		salt and pepper to taste

Bring a medium saucepan of water to a boil over high heat. Add the diced tofu and the turmeric, let the water return to a boil, then cook for 5 minutes. Drain and cool.

Combine the cooled tofu cubes with the celery, onion, mayonnaise and mustard in a bowl. Toss to combine, then season with salt and pepper to taste.

Makes 3 or 4 servings.

Variations

- *Omit the onion, and add a bit of diced apple and some chopped almonds.*
- *Add a dollop of sweet pickle relish or some chopped dill pickles.*

Tofu—it's inevitable.

Now you really have to come to terms with tofu. (If you already have, you can skip this introductory lecture, and move on to the next paragraph.) If you haven't, then don't go anywhere. Tofu is a perfectly harmless substance made from soy beans, which can be used as a highly nutritious alternative to meat. Some non-vegetarians think it's yucky. You can't afford to think that way. Tofu comes in many different forms, and can be prepared in a gazillion different ways, quite a few of them completely undetectable to the naked eye. So, anyone who says tofu is yucky doesn't know what they're talking about. Keep reading.

Tofu is to beans what cheese is to milk. It's the solid protein part of the soy bean, which has been prepared in such a way as to make it versatile and easy to cook. Tofu is available in varying degrees of firmness, from really soft (almost like pudding) to quite hard (like Cheddar cheese). Although a particular recipe may call for a specific type of tofu, you can almost always substitute one type for another in any recipe (with a few exceptions). Some people like the chewy texture of a really firm tofu, while others enjoy the soft, slippery stuff. Whatever.

Tofu is an excellent source of protein, with no cholesterol and very little fat.

Tofu itself is bland and almost tasteless. But it has a remarkable chameleon-like ability to blend into its surroundings and absorb whatever flavors happen to be in the neighborhood. You can marinate it, if you want, or just stir fry it with vegetables and seasonings. Extra firm tofu can be cut into fingers and breaded, turning it into something like fish sticks (without the fish). Squishy tofu can be blended into a sauce like mayonnaise. If you freeze tofu, then thaw it out, you can squeeze the water out of it by hand and crumble it into an amazingly meat-like substance, which can then be thrown into chili, spaghetti sauce, or turned into burgers. How can anyone say this is yucky stuff? Like, what part, exactly, is yucky?

Now no one is telling you to eat tofu every single day. Although you could. And no one is saying you will love everything you make with it. I mean, even chocolate has its bad moments. But if you're a vegetarian, tofu is certainly worth messing around with until you get it right.

All we are saying, is give tofu a chance.

Couscous Salad

Add whatever odds and ends of vegetables you have in the house. This is a very flexible salad.

1 cup	250 mL	water
1 cup	250 mL	dry couscous
4		green onions, chopped
2		medium cucumbers, diced
2		medium green peppers, chopped
1		(19-oz./540 mL) can beans, any kind—black, kidney, pinto, chick-peas, drained (2 cups/500 mL home-cooked)
½ cup	125 mL	chopped fresh parsley
2 tbsp.	30 mL	lemon juice
¼ cup	50 mL	olive oil
½ tsp.	2 mL	ground cumin
		salt and pepper to taste
		and, really, whatever else you like: canned baby corn, sun-dried tomatoes, hot peppers, chocolate chips (just kidding)

In a medium saucepan, bring the water to a boil, stir in the couscous, then immediately remove from heat and cover the pot. Let the couscous stand, covered, for 5 or 10 minutes, while you prepare the other ingredients. The couscous will absorb all the liquid. Fluff gently with a fork to loosen.

In a very large bowl, combine all the vegetables and the parsley with the cooked couscous. Mix gently, making sure you don't mash up the ingredients.

In an empty jar, combine the lemon juice, oil and cumin. Screw on the lid, and shake to mix. Pour this dressing over the couscous and toss. Add salt and pepper to taste, cover the bowl and chill until serving time. If there doesn't seem to be enough dressing, you can add a bit more olive oil and another squirt of lemon juice.

Makes 8 or 10 servings.

Pasta Salad

Great to take on a picnic because it contains nothing that will turn scary in the heat. For eating in the safety of your own home, however, you can toss in a couple of hard-cooked eggs cut into wedges, if you like.

4 cups	1 L	rotini (or other medium-sized) pasta
1 tbsp.	15 mL	vegetable oil
2 cups	500 mL	broccoli flowerets, very lightly steamed
1		small zucchini, sliced and lightly steamed
3		medium tomatoes, diced
1 cup	250 mL	snow peas, halved and blanched
¼ cup	50 mL	chopped onion
¼ cup	50 mL	chopped fresh parsley
2 tbsp.	30 mL	chopped fresh basil
¼ cup	50 mL	olive or vegetable oil
2 tbsp.	30 mL	cider or wine vinegar
2 tbsp.	30 mL	grated Parmesan cheese
1		clove garlic, minced
		salt and pepper to taste

Cook the rotini, rinse under cold water and drain thoroughly. Toss it with 1 tbsp./15 mL oil and let it cool while you prepare the rest of the ingredients. When the pasta is cold, add the broccoli, zucchini, tomatoes, snow peas, onion, parsley and basil. Toss well to combine. Refrigerate, covered, until serving time.

In a small bowl, whisk together the oil, vinegar, Parmesan cheese, garlic, and salt and pepper. *Just before serving*, pour the dressing over the salad, and toss to coat everything. Don't add the dressing too far ahead of time, because it will soak into the pasta and disappear.

Makes 4 to 6 servings.

Gazillion Bean Salad

If you want an almost instant salad, use three cans of mixed beans. Most mixtures will contain red and white kidney beans, chick-peas, romano beans or black-eyed peas. Very colorful.

3		(19-oz./540 mL) cans any kind of beans, drained (6 cups/1.5 L home-cooked)
1		medium red or yellow onion, chopped
1		medium sweet green or red pepper, chopped
1		medium tomato, diced
¼ cup	50 mL	chopped fresh parsley (or cilantro for a Mexican touch)
½ cup	125 mL	olive or vegetable oil
⅓ cup	75 mL	cider vinegar
1		clove garlic, squished
2 tbsp.	30 mL	sugar
1 tsp.	5 mL	salt
½ tsp.	2 mL	pepper

In a large bowl, toss together the beans, onion, sweet pepper, tomato and parsley.

In a small bowl whisk together the oil, vinegar, garlic, sugar, salt and pepper. Pour this dressing over the bean mixture, cover, and chill for at least 1 hour. Toss salad again just before serving.

Makes 6 to 8 servings.

Wild and Brown Rice Salad

Serve this wonderful salad with some oven-roasted vegetables and a loaf of good bread for a great fall dinner.

½ cup	125 mL	raw wild rice
1 cup	250 mL	raw brown rice
1		medium red onion, chopped
1		medium sweet red or yellow pepper, chopped
2		stalks celery, thinly sliced
2 tbsp.	30 mL	chopped fresh parsley
¼ cup	50 mL	chopped pecans, lightly toasted
2 tbsp.	30 mL	orange juice
2 tbsp.	30 mL	lemon juice
1 tsp.	5 mL	orange rind
1 tsp.	5 mL	lemon rind
⅓ cup	75 mL	olive or vegetable oil

First, in separate saucepans, cook the wild and brown rice. See rice-cooking basics on page 168 for detailed instructions. Let rice cool to room temperature.

Combine the wild and brown rice in a large bowl. Add the onion, sweet pepper, celery, parsley and pecans. Toss lightly to mix.

In a small bowl, whisk together the orange and lemon juices and rind, and the olive oil. Pour over the rice mixture in the bowl, and toss.

Makes 4 to 6 servings.

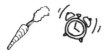# Zingy Carrot Salad

In the middle of winter, when even the most depressing head of lettuce costs a fortune, make a colorful carrot salad instead. It's guaranteed to cheer you up. For a hearty fall feast, serve this with Split Pea Soup (page 41), Zucchini and Basil Strata (page 88) and Fruit Compote (page 205).

6		medium carrots, peeled or scrubbed and shredded
¼ cup	50 mL	lemon juice
¼ cup	50 mL	olive or vegetable oil
1 tsp.	5 mL	Dijon mustard
½ tsp.	2 mL	salt

Plus optional ingredients (choose one or more):

1		clove garlic, squished
¼ tsp.	1 mL	hot pepper sauce
½ cup	125 mL	sunflower seed kernels
¼ cup	50 mL	chopped fresh parsley
¼ cup	50 mL	chopped fresh coriander
2 tbsp.	30 mL	chopped fresh mint
½ cup	125 mL	raisins
1 tsp.	5 mL	caraway seeds
½ tsp.	2 mL	ground cumin seeds

Toss together the shredded carrots, lemon juice, oil, mustard and salt. Add optional ingredients of your choice and mix well.

   Makes 3 or 4 servings.

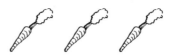

Taboulleh

This is a recipe for a classic taboulleh. If you want, you can toss in a can of drained chick-peas to turn it into a full meal.

1 cup	250 mL	uncooked bulgur wheat
3 cups	750 mL	boiling water
3		tomatoes, diced
3		green onions, chopped
½ cup	125 mL	fresh parsley, chopped
½ cup	125 mL	fresh mint, chopped (or you can omit the mint and use all parsley)
¼ cup	50 mL	olive oil
2 tbsp.	30 mL	lemon juice (preferably fresh)
1		clove garlic (or more, or less—you decide), squished
½ tsp.	2 mL	salt
¼ tsp.	1 mL	pepper
1		cucumber, thinly sliced

Measure the bulgur wheat into a large mixing bowl, add the boiling water and stir. Let it sit, and absorb the water, while you prepare the rest of the ingredients— at least 15 minutes.

Chop the tomatoes, green onions, parsley and mint. Combine in a large bowl.

In a small bowl or measuring cup, mix together the olive oil, lemon juice, garlic, salt and pepper. Set aside.

By this time, the bulgur should be finished soaking. Line a strainer or a colander with a dish towel, dump the bulgur into it and, twisting the corners of the towel together, squeeze as much of the water out as you can. The bulgur should be fluffy and soft, but not soggy. Add to the vegetable mixture in the large bowl. Stir in the dressing, and toss very well.

To serve, mound the taboulleh on a platter or bowl, and decorate with cucumber slices.

Makes 4 to 6 servings.

Spicy Oriental Asparagus Salad

Addictive. You can't stop eating it.

1½ lbs.	750 g	fresh asparagus, trimmed and cut into 2-inch (5 cm) pieces
1 tbsp.	15 mL	Chinese chili paste
2 tbsp.	30 mL	sugar
2 tbsp.	30 mL	vinegar
2 tbsp.	30 mL	sesame oil
1 tsp.	5 mL	salt
3 tbsp.	45 mL	vegetable oil
6		cloves garlic, cut into slivers

Chinese Chili Paste

There are many kinds of Chinese chili paste—some made with garlic, others that include beans. They all contain crushed chilies and vegetable oil and are quite spicy. For most purposes, you can use chili paste with garlic. It comes in a jar and can be found in Chinese grocery stores and some large supermarkets. A dash of hot pepper sauce can be used as a substitute.

Place asparagus pieces in a steamer basket over boiling water and steam for 2 or 3 minutes—just until they go bright green, but before they begin to get soft. Dump into a strainer, and run cold water over to stop them from cooking further. Let them drain.

In a small bowl, combine the chili paste, sugar, vinegar, sesame oil and salt. Set aside.

In a wok or large skillet, heat the vegetable oil over high heat. Add the garlic slivers, stir-fry for no more than 1 minute, then add the chili paste mixture. Remove from heat and add the asparagus, tossing to combine well.

Chill completely before serving. If you can wait that long.

Makes 1 serving. Just kidding. Maybe 4.

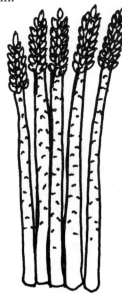

Dynamic Dressings
Basic Vinaigrette Dressing

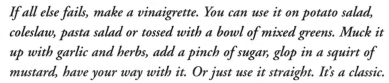

If all else fails, make a vinaigrette. You can use it on potato salad, coleslaw, pasta salad or tossed with a bowl of mixed greens. Muck it up with garlic and herbs, add a pinch of sugar, glop in a squirt of mustard, have your way with it. Or just use it straight. It's a classic.

½ cup	125 mL	olive or vegetable oil
¼ cup	50 mL	vinegar
		salt and pepper to taste

Combine all the ingredients in a jar, and shake until mixed. That's it.

Now go ahead and do something with it.

Makes ¾ cup (175 mL) dressing.

Variations on the theme

- *Add 1 tsp. (5 mL) Dijon mustard.*
- *Add a squished clove of garlic.*
- *Sprinkle in a bit of sugar to cut the acidity.*
- *Use some of that fancy walnut or hazelnut oil you got from Aunt Doris last Christmas.*
- *Blend in a bit of mayonnaise to make it creamy.*
- *Try red or white wine vinegar, cider vinegar, a flavored vinegar or lemon juice instead.*
- *Add a pinch of whatever fresh or dried herbs you think might work.*
- *Add a squirt of ketchup (really).*
- *Sprinkle in some Parmesan cheese.*

Sun-Dried Tomato Vinaigrette Dressing

Olive Oil

A person could spend a lot of money on olive oil. But you don't have to. In salad dressings or anywhere that the flavor of the olive oil will actually matter, use extra virgin olive oil—the best you can afford. The words "extra virgin" on the label mean that the oil has been extracted without the use of heat, and you can be pretty sure it will have a nice olive flavor. For cooking purposes—like for sautéing vegetables or in spicy sauces—you can get away with ordinary olive oil (usually labeled "pure olive oil"), which is considerably cheaper.

What a nifty salad dressing. Colorful and delicious, it keeps almost indefinitely in the refrigerator, and is perfect on a mixed green salad.

¼ cup	50 mL	sun-dried tomatoes (packed in oil), chopped
2 tbsp.	30 mL	minced onion
1 or 2		cloves garlic, chopped
½ tsp.	2 mL	salt
¼ tsp.	1 mL	pepper
¼ cup	50 mL	white wine or apple cider vinegar
1 tbsp.	15 mL	water
½ cup	125 mL	olive oil
½ cup	125 mL	vegetable oil

Dump all the ingredients except the olive and vegetable oils into the container of a blender or food processor. Blend until the tomatoes are minced, then scrape down the sides of the container and replace the lid. Turn the blender or processor back on and add the oils through the small opening in the lid, pouring them in a thin stream, while the motor is running. Blend until the dressing is thickened.

Makes about 2 cups (500 mL).

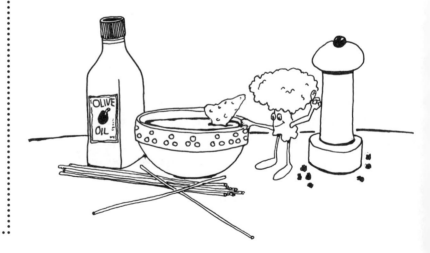

Balsamic Garlic Dressing

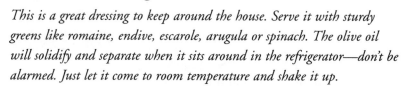

This is a great dressing to keep around the house. Serve it with sturdy greens like romaine, endive, escarole, arugula or spinach. The olive oil will solidify and separate when it sits around in the refrigerator—don't be alarmed. Just let it come to room temperature and shake it up.

1 cup	250 mL	olive oil
¼ cup	50 mL	balsamic vinegar
1 tbsp.	15 mL	Dijon mustard
2		cloves garlic, chopped
1 tsp.	5 mL	salt
1 tsp.	5 mL	pepper

In a blender or food processor, blend all the ingredients together until emulsified. Store whatever you don't use immediately in a jar in the refrigerator.

Makes about 1½ cups (375 mL).

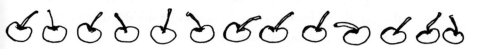

Creamy Greek Dressing

This is great to use on green salad, or with tomatoes, cucumbers and feta cheese. Keep any leftover dressing refrigerated. Let it come to room temperature before serving.

¼ cup	50 mL	lemon juice
¼ cup	50 mL	white wine or apple cider vinegar
2 tsp.	10 mL	crumbled dried oregano
1½ tsp.	7 mL	salt
1½ tsp.	7 mL	sugar
½ tsp.	2 mL	pepper
6		cloves garlic (yes, really)
1½ cups	375 mL	olive or vegetable oil (or a mixture of both)

Into the container of a blender or food processor, measure the lemon juice, vinegar, oregano, salt, sugar, pepper and garlic cloves. Blend until everything is pulverized. Scrape down the sides, then replace the lid. Now, turn the machine back on and add the oil in a thin stream, pouring it in through the small opening in the lid while the motor is running. Keep blending until the dressing is thickened and creamy.

Makes about 2 cups (500 mL).

Garlic

Garlic has long been known to possess medicinal properties. It has been used to ward off disease and vampires, and serious devotees will even wear a string of garlic around their necks for personal protection. How can you not love something like that? When shopping for garlic, look for the largest heads of garlic you can find, with big, firm cloves (the individual sections) with papery white or reddish skin.

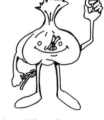

Yogurt Tahini Dressing

When you first make this dressing, it will be creamy and pourable.
Refrigerate it, and it will become thick enough to use as a dip.

1 cup	250 mL	plain yogurt
½ cup	125 mL	tahini
1		clove garlic, squished
2 tbsp.	30 mL	lemon juice
2 tbsp.	30 mL	finely chopped parsley
1 tbsp.	15 mL	finely chopped green onion
½ tsp.	2 mL	salt

In a medium bowl, or in a blender or food processor, mix together all
the ingredients, stirring (or blending) until fairly smooth.

Serve with mixed green or tomato and cucumber salad, as a dip
with fresh vegetables, or spoon it into a veggie-stuffed pita sandwich.

Makes about 1¾ cups (425 mL) dressing.

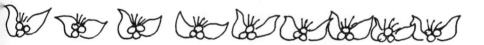

Tofu Mayonnaise

Okay, so it's not exactly identical to normal mayo, but still. For most purposes, this eggless version of mayonnaise can be used instead of the regular kind. So yes, go ahead, have a dab of mayo on your sandwich.

½ lb.	250 g	regular tofu (about 2 medium squares)
¼ cup	50 mL	lemon juice
2 tsp.	10 mL	Dijon mustard
1 tsp.	5 mL	salt
1 tsp.	5 mL	sugar
1 cup	250 mL	vegetable oil

With a fork or with your bare hands, mash the tofu and place it in a strainer or colander set over a bowl. Weight it down slightly with a plate or bowl and allow the excess liquid to drain out for about half an hour.

Place the drained tofu into the container of a blender or food processor. Add the lemon juice, mustard, salt and sugar, and blend, scraping down the sides of the container once or twice, until smooth. Now, replace the lid on the container and, with the motor running, pour the oil in through the small opening in the lid very gradually. Stop the machine and scrape down the sides of the container once or twice so that the mixture blends evenly.

Tofu mayonnaise will keep, refrigerated, for about a week.

Makes about 2 cups (500 mL).

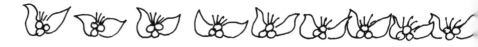

5. Exceptional Eggs and Perfect Pancakes

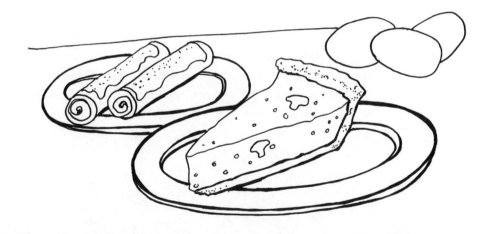

Exceptional Eggs Whole Wheat Buttermilk French Toast

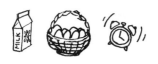

Great for breakfast but even better as a midnight snack.

2		eggs
¼ cup	50 mL	buttermilk
1 tbsp.	15 mL	sugar
1 tsp.	5 mL	vanilla extract
4 to 6		slices homemade-style whole wheat bread
2 tbsp.	30 mL	vegetable oil

In a flat dish—like a pie plate—beat together the eggs, buttermilk, sugar and vanilla. Dip the bread slices into the egg mixture, turning to coat both sides. Don't let the bread linger in the bowl too long or it will soak up all the egg mixture—a quick dip will do.

Heat the oil in a skillet over medium heat. When the oil is hot, add as many slices as will fit in the pan without crowding and cook until golden brown. Turn and cook the other side and serve immediately. With maple syrup, of course.

Makes 2 servings.

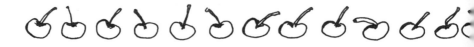

Scrambled Tofu

This is great rolled into a tortilla (with a sploosh of salsa, of course), or as a filling for pita pockets. Also good on a plate with a toasted bagel and the Sunday crossword.

1 tbsp.	15 mL	vegetable oil or butter
½		small onion, chopped
½		green or red sweet pepper, chopped
½ lb.	250 g	regular tofu (about 2 medium squares), cut into ¼-inch (.5 cm) dice
¼ tsp.	2 mL	turmeric
¼ tsp.	2 mL	paprika
		salt and pepper to taste

Heat the vegetable oil or butter in a small skillet over medium heat. Add the onion and sweet pepper and cook, stirring once in a while, until soft—8 to 10 minutes. Add the diced tofu, the turmeric and paprika, and cook stirring and mashing slightly, for 5 or 6 minutes, or until heated through and scrambled-looking. Season with salt and pepper to taste.

Makes 2 servings.

Power-Packed Fruit Smoothie

Don't droop. Drink this and feel all new again. A pretty good breakfast too.

1 cup	250 mL	silken tofu (about half of a 19-oz./ 539 g vacuum package)
1		medium banana
2 cups	500 mL	orange juice
1 cup	250 mL	canned unsweetened crushed pineapple

Combine all the ingredients in a blender and blend until smooth. Serve immediately.

Makes about 3 servings.

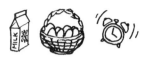

Fast Frittata

A couple of mushrooms, three stalks of asparagus, an old onion, a withered potato. Can this possibly be dinner? You bet.

¼ cup	50 mL	olive or vegetable oil
1		medium onion, chopped
1½ cups	375 mL	sliced or diced vegetables—raw mushrooms, zucchini, peppers, spinach, asparagus, cooked potato, green beans, corn, carrots, broccoli—use your imagination
6		eggs, beaten
¼ cup	50 mL	grated Parmesan cheese
		chopped fresh herbs (if you have them)
		salt and pepper to taste
2 tbsp.	30 mL	butter or margarine

Heat the oil in a 10-inch (25 cm) skillet over medium heat. Add the chopped onion and cook, stirring, for about 5 minutes, until the onion is softened. Throw in whatever raw vegetables you're using and cook until they're almost tender, then stir in any cooked vegetables and sauté for 1 or 2 minutes longer, until everything is heated through.

Remove the vegetable mixture from the skillet and add to the beaten eggs in a bowl. Stir in 2 tbsp. (30 mL) of the grated Parmesan cheese, whatever herbs you're using, and salt and pepper to taste. Stir to combine.

Melt the butter over medium heat in the same skillet in which you cooked the vegetables. Let it get foamy, then pour in the egg and vegetable mixture, spreading it evenly in the pan. Lower the heat to very low and cook, gently, for 15 to 20 minutes, just until the eggs are set but still wobbly in the middle.

Sprinkle the frittata with the remaining Parmesan cheese and place under a preheated broiler element for 1 to 2 minutes, just until the top is set and lightly browned.

Loosen the edges of the frittata with a knife and slide it out onto a plate. Cut into wedges to serve.

Makes 3 to 4 servings.

Quickie Quiche

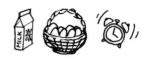

A quiche can elevate a humble mess of leftover vegetable odds and ends into a delicious main dish. A little of this and a little of that—and it's supper.

2 tbsp.	30 mL	vegetable oil
½		medium onion, chopped
1½ cups	375 mL	prepared vegetables (see below)
2 cups	500 mL	shredded Swiss or Cheddar cheese
3		eggs
1 cup	250 mL	plain yogurt (or milk or soy milk)
		salt and pepper to taste
1		unbaked 9-inch (22 cm) pie shell, home-made or store-bought

Heat the vegetable oil in a medium skillet over medium heat. Add the onion and cook, stirring, until tender—6 to 8 minutes. Stir in the prepared vegetables and, if they're raw, cook until just tender. If the vegetables are already cooked, sauté them for a couple of minutes to heat through and combine with the onion. Let cool for a minute, then spread over the bottom of the pie crust and sprinkle with the shredded cheese.

In a small bowl, beat together the eggs and the yogurt (or milk). Add salt and pepper to taste, and pour over the vegetables and cheese.

Bake at 375° F (190° C) for 35 to 40 minutes, until puffed and golden. A knife inserted into the middle of the quiche should come out clean.

Makes 4 to 6 servings.

Just a Few Quiche Possibilities

- *Sliced mushrooms*
- *Sliced zucchini*
- *Chopped cooked spinach*
- *Chopped cooked green beans*
- *Broccoli flowerets*
- *Chopped asparagus*
- *Shredded carrots*
- *Chopped tomatoes*

Zucchini and Basil Strata

No zucchini? Make this with chopped fresh spinach or broccoli instead.

6 cups	1.5 L	bread cubes (preferably stale)
2 cups	500 mL	chopped zucchini
1 cup	250 mL	shredded Swiss cheese
6		eggs
2 cups	500 mL	milk
¼ cup	50 mL	chopped fresh basil (or 1 tbsp./15 mL dried)
¼ tsp.	1 mL	ground nutmeg
		salt and pepper to taste

In a greased 8-cup (2 L) casserole, layer half the bread cubes, half the zucchini, and half the Swiss cheese, sprinkling each layer with salt and pepper. Repeat layers, ending with cheese.

Beat the eggs with the milk, basil and nutmeg. Pour the egg mixture over the bread, zucchini and cheese layers. Cover with plastic wrap and refrigerate at least 2 hours or overnight.

Bake, uncovered, at 350° F (180° C) for 45 to 55 minutes, until puffed and set in the center.

Makes 6 to 8 servings.

Baked Broccoli + Egg Squares

This is sort of like a quiche without a crust. It's the kind of thing that you can make with whatever vegetable you have around instead of the fresh broccoli—zucchini, cauliflower, cooked leftover potatoes or even a mixture of vegetables. And if you don't have any fresh vegetables at all, you can use an equal amount of frozen (you won't need to cook those, just defrost them).

4 cups	1 litre	chopped fresh broccoli (1 medium bunch, stalks and flowerets chopped separately)
5		eggs
2 tbsp.	30 mL	flour
½ tsp.	2 mL	baking powder
1 cup	250 mL	shredded Swiss or Cheddar cheese
½ tsp.	2 mL	salt
¼ tsp.	1 mL	pepper

Place the chopped broccoli stalks in a steamer basket over boiling water and steam for 5 minutes, then add the flowerets and steam for another 3 minutes. Dump broccoli into a greased 8-inch (20 cm) square baking dish, spreading it out to cover the bottom evenly.

In a medium bowl, beat the eggs with the flour and baking powder just until smooth, then stir in the cottage cheese. Pour egg mixture over the broccoli in the baking dish. Bake at 350° F (180° C) for 25 minutes, sprinkle with shredded cheese and bake for another 3 to 5 minutes, until the center is almost set and the cheese is melted.

Makes about 6 servings.

Perfect Pancakes

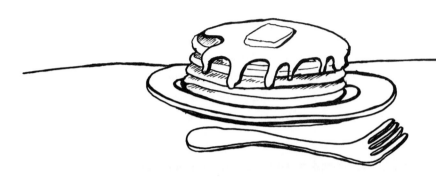

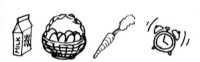 ## Fluffy Pancakes

These pancakes are so light and fluffy, you may have to glue them down to your plate with maple syrup so that they don't float away.

1 cup	250 mL	all-purpose flour
2 tbsp.	30 mL	sugar
2 tbsp.	30 mL	baking powder
1		egg
1 cup	250 mL	milk
2 tbsp.	30 mL	oil

In a medium bowl, combine the flour, sugar and baking powder. Yes, that *is* 2 tablespoons (30 mL) of baking powder.

In a small bowl, whisk together the egg, milk and oil, then add to the dry ingredients and beat until smooth.

Heat an oiled griddle or frying pan and pour in the batter, about ¼ cup (50 mL) at a time. Allow pancakes to cook on one side until bubbles appear on the top, then flip and let the other side cook until golden.

Makes about 12 four-inch (10 cm) pancakes.

Whole Wheat Buttermilk Pancakes

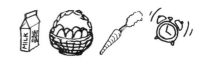

A classic. Even better with some blueberries thrown in.

1¼ cup	300 mL	whole wheat flour
1 tbsp.	30 mL	sugar
1 tsp.	5 mL	baking powder
½ tsp.	2 mL	baking soda
1¼ cup	300 mL	buttermilk (or see substitutes)
1		egg
2 tbsp.	30 mL	oil

In a large bowl stir together the flour, sugar, baking powder and baking soda until well mixed. Pour in the buttermilk, egg and oil and whisk until smooth.

Heat an oiled griddle or frying pan and pour in the batter, ¼ cup (50 mL) at a time, spreading it into an even layer. If the batter is too thick to pour easily, add a little more milk to thin it.

Allow pancakes to cook on one side until bubbles appear on the top, then flip and let the other side cook until golden.

Makes about 12 four-inch (10 cm) pancakes.

Buttermilk Substitutes

- *Use plain yogurt thinned with a little milk.*
- *Stir 1 tbsp. (15 mL) vinegar into the milk in the recipe and let it sit at room temperature for 10 minutes to sour. It will curdle—don't be alarmed—it's perfectly normal.*

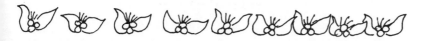

Plain Crepes

Once you get the hang of making crepes, you'll think of a million things to do with them. Stuff them with sautéed mushrooms, or steamed asparagus, or spinach. Roll them around the same filling that goes into the Broccoli-stuffed Pasta Shells (page 116). Serve them for dessert—filled with fresh fruit or ice cream or something chocolate.

1 cup	250 mL	flour
2		eggs
1¾ cups	400 mL	milk
½ tsp.	2 mL	salt (if using for savory dishes) *or*
1 tsp.	5 mL	sugar (if using for sweet dishes)

Measure all ingredients into a blender, and blend until smooth. Let batter stand, covered and refrigerated, for at least 1 hour before using. (This standing time allows the batter to thicken slightly and makes it easier to work with.)

Brush an 8- to 10-inch (20 to 25 cm) nonstick frying pan lightly with vegetable oil, and place over medium heat until a drop of water sizzles when it hits the pan. Pour in about ¼ cup (50 mL) of crepe batter, swirling the pan around to coat the bottom evenly. This takes some practice, so don't feel bad if the first few crepes turn out very weird.

When the top of the crepe starts to look a bit dry and the bottom is just beginning to brown (peek underneath to check), flip the crepe over with a thin-bladed spatula. Cook for just 30 seconds, then turn out onto a plate—cover and keep warm if you'll be using them right away. Brush the pan again lightly with oil, and repeat the process until you have used up all of the batter.

Makes 10 to 12 crepes, if all goes well.

Leftover crepes (as if that would happen!) can be wrapped in plastic and frozen. Just defrost, fill and reheat in the oven.

Creative Crepe Fillings

Here are just a few suggestions for things you can roll into a crepe—for both savory dishes or desserts. But don't feel limited to these ideas—you can fill a crepe with just about anything at all, or even have them plain with a squirt of lemon juice and a sprinkle of sugar. There is simply no bad way to eat a crepe.

SAVORY

- Sliced mushrooms sautéed in butter, with a slosh of cream, a sprinkle of Parmesan, and seasoned with parsley, salt and pepper.
- Ratatouille (page 178).
- Sautéed sweet peppers, onions and tomatoes and shredded Cheddar cheese.

- Steamed broccoli, sprinkled with lemon juice, salt and pepper and shredded Swiss cheese.
- Fill with the broccoli and ricotta cheese mixture from Broccoli Stuffed Shells (page 116), place in a baking dish, cover and bake for a few minutes until heated through.

SWEET

- Sliced apples, sautéed in butter with sugar, cinnamon and lemon juice.
- Peach and banana flambé mixture (page 206) served with ice cream on the side.

- Fresh strawberries, raspberries, blueberries or peaches, sweetened with maple syrup and served with whipped cream.
- Apricot or strawberry jam.

- Fill with a mixture of cream cheese or ricotta cheese, lightly sweetened, and flavored with a squirt of vanilla extract. Place in a baking dish, dot with butter and bake for a few minutes until heated through. Serve with fresh or defrosted frozen berries, sweetened with a bit of maple syrup or honey.

- Ice cream. And chocolate sauce.

6. Marvelous Main Dishes

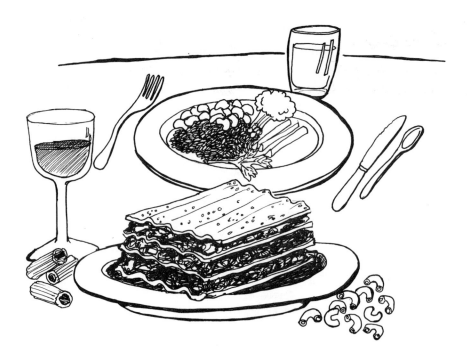

Positively Pastas and Splendid Sauces

All-Purpose Tomato Pasta Sauce

Everyone needs a good old reliable spaghetti sauce up their sleeve. This recipe makes a nice big batch and can be used on pasta, to make lasagne or pizza, in any recipe that calls for plain spaghetti sauce.

2 tbsp.	30 mL	olive or vegetable oil
1		onion, chopped
2 or 3		cloves garlic, squished
1		carrot, finely chopped
1		stalk celery, finely chopped
8 cups	2 L	chopped fresh tomatoes (or two 19-oz./796 mL cans)
2 tbsp.	30 mL	tomato paste
1 tsp.	5 mL	salt
½ tsp.	2 mL	pepper
1 tsp.	5 mL	crumbled dried oregano
¼ cup	50 mL	chopped fresh parsley or basil (or some of each)

In a large pot or Dutch oven, heat the oil over medium heat. Add the onion and garlic and cook, stirring, for about 5 minutes, or until the onion is transparent. Add the carrot and celery, and continue to cook for another 6 to 8 minutes, until the vegetables are beginning to soften. Dump in the tomatoes (if you are using canned tomatoes, don't drain them), the tomato paste, the salt, pepper, oregano and parsley or basil. Bring to a boil, then lower the heat and let simmer, stirring occasionally, until the sauce is thickened—35 to 45 minutes. Taste for seasoning, and add whatever you think it needs.

Use immediately, spooned over hot pasta, or freeze to use any time you need a plain spaghetti sauce. If you prefer a smooth texture, run the finished sauce through a food mill or food processor before using.

Makes about 5 cups (1.25 L).

Have it Your Way!

You can turn this plain spaghetti sauce into something more closely resembling, you know, meat sauce by adding some rehydrated TVP (texturized vegetable protein), crumbled tempeh or commercial hamburger substitute to the pot with the carrot and celery at the beginning of the recipe. Or, for a more veggie-loaded sauce, add some sautéed mushrooms, zucchini or peppers near the end of the cooking time.

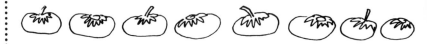

Yes! You Can Freeze Tomatoes!

You have somehow come into a bushel of tomatoes. Okay, so you eat lots of tomato salads. And you make some spaghetti sauce. What do you do with the rest? Well, freeze them.

Nothing could be easier than freezing tomatoes. Pack them into plastic bags and throw them in the freezer. That's pretty much it. When you want to use them, take out as many as you need and run them under hot water for a few seconds. The peels will slip right off. Don't use them raw, though—they'll be mushy and weird. But cooked, they're just great.

Perfect Pesto Sauce

Get your hands on a big bunch of fresh basil, and make lots of this dynamite pesto to use right now or stash away in the freezer. You'll be so happy you did.

¼ cup	50 mL	pine nuts
½ cup	125 mL	olive oil
2 cups	500 mL	fresh basil leaves
2		cloves garlic (or more, whatever…)
½ tsp.	2 mL	salt
¾ cup	175 mL	grated Parmesan cheese (freshly grated if possible)

In a small skillet over medium-low heat, toast the pine nuts in 1 tbsp. (15 mL) of the olive oil—stirring constantly just until they begin to turn golden. Be very careful not to let the pine nuts burn. Toasting the pine nuts really brings out their flavor.

Dump the toasted pine nuts into the bowl of a food processor and add the rest of the olive oil, the basil leaves, garlic and salt. Process until almost (but not quite totally) smooth, scraping down the sides of the bowl a couple of times so that the sauce blends evenly. Add the Parmesan cheese and process just to mix.

That's it.

Makes about 2 cups (500 mL) or enough to toss with 4 servings of pasta, with enough left over to freeze.

Plenty of Other Pestobilities

- Whisk into a Basic Vinaigrette Dressing (page 77) for a pesto vinaigrette.
- Dab onto squares of Grilled Polenta (page 141) and top with a sliver of sun-dried tomato.
- Add a spoonful to Minestrone Soup (page 48).
- Stir into a mixture of yogurt and mayonnaise for a delicious dip.

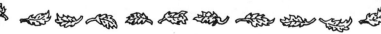

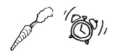

Roasted Tomato Fettuccine

Imagine a pasta sauce that actually cooks itself. This is it. Try this accompanied by a tossed green salad (page 58), Fabulous Focaccia (page 190) and Truly Astonishing Tofu Chocolate Mousse (page 207).

2 lb.	1 kg	ripe plum tomatoes (8 to 10 medium)
¼ cup	50 mL	olive oil
4		cloves garlic, chopped
¼ cup	50 mL	chopped fresh basil leaves
1 tsp.	5 mL	salt
1 lb.	500 g	fettuccine
		grated Parmesan cheese (optional)
		pepper to taste

Cut the stem end off each tomato, then cut them lengthwise into quarters (or sixths, if they're large). Place in a bowl and toss with the olive oil and chopped garlic. Spread tomatoes out in one layer on a large cookie sheet or baking pan. Roast at 400° F (200° C) for 35 to 40 minutes, until they are all squishy and the skins are starting to wrinkle. Don't stir or turn them at all while they're cooking.

Place the chopped basil and the salt in a large bowl.

Meanwhile, cook your pasta in plenty of boiling, salted water, timing it so that the pasta and the tomatoes will be done at the exact same moment. Well, *try*, anyway.

When the tomatoes are done, scoop them directly into the bowl with the basil, gently scraping the bottom of the baking pan to get all the juices and some of that nice burnt stuff too. Add the drained pasta, and toss to mix. Add some pepper and more salt, if necessary, and sprinkle with grated Parmesan cheese.

Makes 4 wonderfully tomatoey servings.

Pasta with Sun-Dried Tomatoes

This is a wonderful, quick tomato sauce with an intense tomato flavor—thanks to the sun-dried tomatoes. Use oil-packed sun-dried tomatoes for this dish, and save the oil to sauté the garlic.

1 tbsp.	15 mL	oil drained from a jar of sun-dried tomatoes, or olive oil
4		cloves garlic, squished
3 cups	750 mL	chopped fresh tomatoes (or 19-oz./ 796 mL can, drained)
¾ cup	175 mL	chopped sun-dried tomatoes from a jar, drained
½ cup	125 mL	chopped fresh basil (or 1 tbsp./15 mL dried)
1 cup	250 mL	vegetable broth
½ cup	125 mL	pine nuts
		salt and pepper
1 lb.	500 g	fettuccine, spaghetti or other pasta
		Parmesan cheese (optional)

Bonus Recipe!

Add 2 cups (500 mL) fresh broccoli flowerets to the sauce when you add the tomatoes, and you'll have a slightly different (and very colorful) dish.

In a large saucepan, heat the oil over medium-low heat. Add the garlic, and cook gently for about 5 minutes, until just beginning to turn golden. Add the fresh tomatoes, sun-dried tomatoes and basil. Cook, stirring, for about 5 minutes. Stir in the vegetable broth and cook for another 5 minutes, then add the pine nuts and season to taste with salt and pepper.

Meanwhile, cook the pasta in plenty of boiling salted water until tender. Drain well.

Toss with hot drained pasta and serve immediately, with some Parmesan cheese for sprinkling at the table.

Makes enough sauce for about 1 lb. (500 g) of pasta.

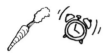

Pasta Puttanesca

This is a great quick pasta sauce that can be thrown together in minutes with stuff from your pantry.

3 tbsp.	45 mL	olive oil
4		cloves garlic, squished
½ cup	125 mL	pitted, chopped brine-cured black olives
2 tbsp.	30 mL	capers
5		large tomatoes (fresh or canned), coarsely chopped
⅓ cup	75 mL	chopped parsley
½ tsp.	2 mL	pepper
½ tsp.	2 mL	red pepper flakes (optional)
1 lb.	500 g	fettuccine or linguine

Heat the olive oil in a large frying pan and add the squished garlic. Cook over low heat for about 5 minutes, until just beginning to color, then add the olives, capers and tomatoes. Cook, stirring, for 10 to 15 minutes, until the sauce is beginning to thicken. Add the parsley, pepper and red pepper flakes (if you're using them).

To serve, cook the pasta in plenty of boiling salted water until tender but firm (al dente), and drain thoroughly. Place about half the sauce in the serving bowl, add the pasta, then top with the rest of the sauce and toss well. This dish is traditionally served *without* cheese (but if you want to add some Parmesan, go ahead).

Makes enough sauce for about 1 lb. (500 g) of pasta.

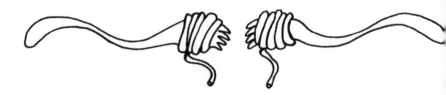

No-Brainer Mushroom Alfredo

Absolutely decadent, perfectly delicious and a total no-brainer.

3 tbsp.	45 mL	butter
1 lb.	500 g	mushrooms, sliced
2		cloves garlic, squished
1½ tbsp.	20 mL	flour
1½ cups	375 mL	milk
½ cup	125 mL	cream cheese, regular or low fat
½ cup	125 mL	grated Parmesan cheese
1 lb.	500 g	fettuccine or linguine
		salt and pepper to taste

Melt the butter in a medium saucepan over medium heat. Add the sliced mushrooms and the garlic, and cook, stirring, until the mushrooms have given up their liquid, and it has evaporated. Sprinkle in the flour, stir, then slowly pour in the milk, stirring constantly. Heat, continuing to stir, until the sauce begins to thicken and just starts to simmer. Add the cream cheese and cook, stirring, until smooth. Remove from heat and stir in the Parmesan cheese.

Meanwhile, cook the fettuccine in plenty of boiling salted water until tender but not mushy. Drain thoroughly, and toss with the mushroom sauce. Season to taste with salt and pepper, and serve immediately.

Makes 4 servings.

Make Too Much Pasta?

Stop! Don't throw out that extra rice or pasta. Just pack it into containers or plastic bags and stash it in the freezer. You can reheat it in a microwave, or thaw it and throw it into soup or a stir-fry.

Fully Loaded Pasta Primavera

This is a stunning, drop-dead pasta dish, best made in spring with the freshest vegetables you can get your mitts on.

1		small zucchini, sliced
1½ cups	375 mL	broccoli flowerets
1½ cups	375 mL	snow peas, cut in half
1 cup	250 mL	fresh or frozen peas
6		stalks asparagus, cut into 1-inch (2 cm) pieces
2 tbsp.	30 mL	olive or vegetable oil
⅓ cup	75 mL	pine nuts
2		cloves garlic, squished
12		cherry tomatoes, cut in half
10		large mushrooms, cut in quarters
⅓ cup	75 mL	butter
1 cup	250 mL	whipping cream
½ cup	125 mL	Parmesan cheese
⅓ cup	75 mL	chopped fresh basil
1 lb.	500 g	spaghetti or fettuccine
		salt and pepper to taste

In a large steamer rack or basket over boiling water, place the zucchini, broccoli, snow peas, regular peas and asparagus. Steam, covered, for about 2 minutes, until just tender-crisp. Rinse under cold running water to stop the cooking, drain thoroughly and set aside.

In a large skillet, heat the olive or vegetable oil. Add the pine nuts and sauté for just a minute or two, until they begin to turn golden. Add the garlic, stir, then add the cherry tomatoes and mushrooms, and cook, stirring, for 1 minute. Now dump in all the steamed vegetables and cook, stirring, for a couple of minutes, until they are heated through.

Meanwhile, in a large saucepan or Dutch oven, melt the butter over medium heat. Add the whipping cream, Parmesan cheese and chopped basil. Stir until the cheese is melted and the sauce is smooth.

Cook the pasta in plenty of boiling salted water until tender but not mushy. Drain well. Pour the cream mixture over the hot spaghetti or fettuccine, toss well, then add about half of the vegetable mixture and toss again. Season to taste with salt and pepper. Dump into a serving bowl and top with the remaining vegetable mixture.

Serve with additional Parmesan cheese.

Makes 4 decadently delicious servings.

Pasta Pointers

For one serving of pasta:

- Long pasta, like spaghetti, fettuccine, etc.—¾-inch (2 cm) diameter bunch

- Medium-sized macaroni shapes (like elbows, small shells, fusilli)—1 cup (250 mL)

- Large-sized macaroni shapes (like rotini, rigatoni, large shells)—1½ cups (375 mL)

- Egg noodles (or other cut noodles)—1⅔ cups (400 mL)

Unscientific Shortcut:

Macaroni will approximately double in volume when cooked. So figure out what size bowl you'll want to end up with, and fill it halfway with dry pasta. That should come out about right.

Another Unscientific Hint:

A 900 g package of pasta will yield about 8 servings as a main dish.

Vegan Alert:

While most Italian-style pasta is made with nothing more than vitamin-enriched flour, *some* varieties do contain traces of egg, and of course, egg noodles will almost certainly contain egg. Get into the habit of checking the label for ingredients.

Pasta à la Caprese

The ultimate midsummer pasta. Make it with the most beautiful, really ripe tomatoes you can find.

8		fresh plum tomatoes, chopped
2		cloves garlic, minced
½		medium red or yellow sweet pepper, chopped
2 tbsp.	30 mL	chopped fresh basil leaves (dried will not do here)
½ cup	125 mL	olive oil
1 tsp.	5 mL	salt
¼ tsp.	1 mL	pepper
1 lb.	500 g	pasta—like shells or penne
2 cups	500 mL	shredded mozzarella cheese
		Parmesan cheese for sprinkling on top

In a bowl, toss together the chopped tomatoes, garlic, sweet pepper, basil, oil, salt and pepper. Let the mixture stand at room temperature for *at least* 1 hour, or as long as 3 hours.

When you're ready to eat, cook the pasta in plenty of boiling salted water until just tender but not mushy. Drain and dump immediately into a large serving bowl. Add the shredded mozzarella cheese and the tomato mixture and toss well.

Serve immediately with Parmesan cheese for sprinkling at the table.

Makes 4 servings.

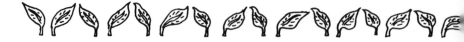

Peculiar Peanut Pasta

Oddly appealing, unusually delicious, amusingly different.

1 tbsp.	15 mL	vegetable oil
2 tbsp.	30 mL	finely chopped onion
1		clove garlic, squished
2 tsp.	10 mL	finely grated ginger root
2		green onions, sliced
1 tsp.	5 mL	Chinese chili paste
1 tbsp.	15 mL	soy sauce
½ tsp.	2 mL	ground coriander
½ tsp.	2 mL	ground cumin
¼ cup	50 mL	smooth peanut butter
¾ cup	175 mL	buttermilk or vegetable broth
1 lb.	500 g	spaghetti or linguine or fettuccine or fresh Chinese noodles

Heat the oil in a small saucepan over medium-low heat. Add the onion, garlic and ginger root and cook, stirring, until the onion is softened—3 to 5 minutes. Stir in the green onions, chili paste, soy sauce, coriander and cumin, and cook for another 2 minutes.

Add the peanut butter, stir until smooth, then add the buttermilk or vegetable broth. Heat through. If the sauce is too thick, add a little more buttermilk or broth to thin it until it is pourable.

Meanwhile, cook the pasta in plenty of boiling, salted water until tender but not mushy. Drain well. Toss the sauce with hot cooked pasta.

Makes enough sauce for about 1 lb. (500 g) pasta.

One Step Beyond ...

Toss the finished pasta with some drained canned baby corn cobs, steamed snow peas, a handful of lightly cooked broccoli flowerets, whatever. Or sprinkle the finished dish with some chopped cilantro or peanuts.

> ### Fresh Ginger Root
>
> Dried, powdered ginger—found in spice racks everywhere—bears absolutely no resemblance to the taste of fresh ginger. This weird, knobby root has a wonderful fresh, almost lemony flavor that has no real substitute. Refrigerated, a hunk of it will keep for a long time.

Bombproof Baked Macaroni Casserole

This one sounds too easy to be any good. One pot, no pre-cooking, totally bombproof. And, yes, it's delicious.

Nitpicky Detail

Most cheese is manufactured using an ingredient called rennet, which is an enzyme taken from the stomach of a calf. If you are concerned about using any animal products whatsoever, buy cheese that has been made with vegetable rennet or look for kosher cheese, which never contains animal rennet.

1		small onion, chopped
1½ cups	375 mL	uncooked elbow macaroni
1 cup	250 mL	cubed Cheddar cheese
1 cup	250 mL	water
1 tsp.	5 mL	salt
		pepper to taste
1		(28-oz./796 mL) can diced tomatoes
1 cup	250 mL	bread crumbs
1 tbsp.	15 mL	butter

Dump all the ingredients except the bread crumbs and butter into a well-greased casserole dish. Yes, everything. Yes, just like that. Stir well. Cover the casserole with a lid (or foil wrap) and bake at 350° F (180° C) for 1 hour. You can lift the lid about halfway though the cooking time and give the mixture a stir, if you like, but it's not necessary.

Meanwhile, melt the butter in a small skillet over medium heat. Add the bread crumbs and cook, stirring, for 8 to 10 minutes, until the crumbs are lightly toasted.

After the casserole has baked for 1 hour, remove the lid and sprinkle the buttered crumbs over top. Return to the oven, place under the broiler element, and broil for 3 to 5 minutes, until browned. (Watch this carefully and do not leave the room!)

Makes 4 bombproof servings.

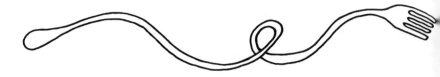

Basic White Sauce
(for just about anything)

You absolutely must know how to make a basic white sauce. It can be tarted up with herbs and spices, turned into a creamy cheese sauce for pasta, or served plain over steamed vegetables. Vegans can use soy milk instead of regular milk—it will turn out just fine.

2 tbsp.	30 mL	butter, margarine or vegetable oil
2 tbsp.	30 mL	all-purpose flour
1 cup	250 mL	milk or soy milk
		salt and pepper to taste

Melt the butter (or margarine or oil) in a small saucepan over low heat. Add the flour, and cook, stirring for just a minute or two. Now slowly add the milk, stirring constantly to eliminate any lumps. Cook, continuing to stir, until the sauce thickens and begins to simmer. Keep cooking the sauce after it reaches a simmer for about 5 minutes, stirring constantly so that it doesn't scorch and stick to the pot.

Season to taste with salt and pepper and, well, that's pretty much it.
Makes 1 cup (250 mL).

Saucy Variations

- Add ½ cup (125 mL) shredded cheese (any kind you like) after removing the sauce from the heat. Stir until smooth and melted.
- Add ½ small onion, minced, to the butter with the flour and cook until soft before adding the milk.
- Stir in ¼ cup (50 mL) chopped parsley or basil to the sauce while it's cooking.
- Make the sauce with vegetable broth instead of milk or soy milk.

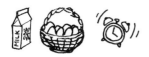

Cheese Noodle Casserole

A deliciously squishy casserole—comforting and creamy, with no weird ingredients or challenging flavors. Perfect for when Aunt Gertrude comes for dinner.

1		(12-oz./340 g) package broad egg noodles
3 tbsp.	45 mL	butter or margarine
2		medium onions, chopped
2		medium carrots, diced
3 tbsp.	45 mL	flour
2 cups	500 mL	milk
2 tbsp.	30 mL	chopped fresh parsley
1 tsp.	5 mL	salt
¼ tsp.	1 mL	pepper
2 tsp.	10 mL	Worcestershire sauce (or soy sauce)
1 cup	250 mL	cottage cheese
1½ cups	375 mL	frozen peas
1 cup	250 mL	shredded Cheddar cheese

Cook the noodles in a large pot of boiling salted water until tender, then rinse under cold running water, and drain thoroughly. Set aside.

In a medium saucepan, melt the butter or margarine, then add the onions and carrots and sauté over medium heat until the carrots begin to soften, 6 to 8 minutes. Stir in the flour and cook for a minute, then add the milk, parsley, salt, pepper and Worcestershire sauce. Cook, stirring almost constantly, until the sauce thickens and gets bubbly. Add the cottage cheese and cook, stirring, just until the cheese melts smoothly into the sauce. Add the peas, let the sauce return to a simmer, then remove from heat.

In a mixing bowl, combine the noodles and sauce and turn the mixture into a greased 2½ quart (2.5 L) casserole dish. Cover and bake at 350° F (180° C) for 25 minutes. Uncover, sprinkle the top with Cheddar cheese, and bake for another 5 to 10 minutes, until the cheese is melted.

Makes 4 to 6 servings.

Soy Milk and Cheese

Soy milk is made from soaked, ground soy beans, which are then strained to produce a liquid that looks pretty much like, well, cow's milk. It can be found either in the refrigerated dairy case of the supermarket (like regular milk), or in an aseptic container (like a juice box) on the shelf (often near the canned milks). It comes in various flavors—chocolate, vanilla, plain—and can be used as a straight substitute for cow's milk in nearly any recipe. You can also, of course, drink it. Or pour it on cereal. Or into your coffee. Or whatever. Soy milk is a good source of protein, and some brands are fortified with B vitamins and/or calcium.

Soy cheese is a rough approximation of regular dairy cheese, and comes in different varieties—to simulate different types of cheese, such as Cheddar and mozzarella. It can be used in much the same way as regular cheese, but the results will vary with the brand—so try several kinds until you find one you like. It's best used where the flavor of the cheese isn't predominant.

Multivegetable Lasagne

This easy lasagne uses oven-ready noodles that don't require pre-cooking. You can substitute other vegetables (broccoli, cauliflower, egg-plant, whatever) if you want, just keep the total amount the same.

¼ cup	50 mL	vegetable or olive oil
1		medium onion, chopped
2		cloves garlic, squished
1 cup	250 mL	coarsely chopped mushrooms
1		small zucchini, diced
1		medium carrot, diced
1		green or red pepper, chopped
4 cups	1 L	spaghetti sauce (28-oz./796 mL can)
1 cup	250 mL	water
2 cups	500 mL	chopped raw spinach
2 cups	500 mL	ricotta or cottage cheese
2		eggs
2 tbsp.	30 mL	chopped fresh parsley
15		oven-ready (no boil) lasagne noodles
3 cups	750 mL	shredded mozzarella cheese
¼ cup	50 mL	grated Parmesan cheese

In a large skillet or saucepan, heat the oil over medium heat. Add the onion and garlic and cook, stirring, for about 5 minutes, until soft-ened. Add the mushrooms, zucchini, carrot and green or red pepper and cook, stirring once in a while, for another 5 to 8 minutes, until the vegetables are beginning to wilt. Now add the spaghetti sauce and the water, lower the heat, and let simmer for about 10 minutes. Toss in the spinach and let cook for 5 minutes longer. Taste and adjust sea-soning with salt and pepper if necessary. Set aside.

In a bowl, mix together the ricotta or cottage cheese, the eggs and the parsley.

Okay—put it together. Spread about 1 cup (250 mL) of the sauce over the bottom of a 9 x 13-inch (22 x 33 cm) baking dish. On this, arrange 5 uncooked lasagne noodles, overlapping them a bit just so they cover the sauce on the bottom of the pan. You may have to break the noodles up just a bit so it all fits. Spread 2 cups (500 mL) of sauce over this, then spoon on half of the ricotta cheese mixture. Sprinkle with 1 cup (250 mL) shredded mozzarella. Repeat layers: 5 noodles, 2 cups (500 mL) sauce, the rest of the ricotta, 1 cup (250 mL) mozzarella. Now finally, top with the last 5 noodles, all the rest of the sauce, and the rest of the mozzarella. Sprinkle the top with Parmesan cheese.

Cover the baking dish loosely with foil and bake at 350° F (180° C) for 30 minutes. Remove the foil and continue baking for another 15 minutes, until the sauce is bubbling and a knife can easily penetrate the lasagne in the middle.

Makes about 8 servings.

Note: You can substitute defrosted crumbled tofu, TVP or crumbled tempeh for a portion of the vegetables in the sauce. Just omit the mushrooms and zucchini, and add 1½ cups (375 mL) of any of the meat substitutes to the sauce instead. Make sure the TVP has been soaked and reconstituted before adding.

Pseudo-Hollandaise Sauce

We've all heard horror stories about how difficult it is to make a proper Hollandaise sauce. So who needs proper? Spoon this easy sauce over hot steamed asparagus, roll it into a crepe with some cooked broccoli or use it as a dip with fresh steamed artichokes.

2		eggs
2 tbsp.	30 mL	lemon juice
¼ tsp.	1 mL	salt
1 cup	250 mL	butter

Place the eggs, lemon juice and salt in the container of a blender.

In a small saucepan, bring the butter to a boil. Remove from heat and immediately add to the ingredients in the blender and blend until foamy.

Makes about 2 cups (500 mL).

Green and White Lasagne

A deliciously different lasagne—perfect for St. Patrick's Day.

12 to 15		lasagne noodles, regular or spinach
10 oz.	284 g	package fresh spinach
15 oz.	475 g	ricotta cheese
4		eggs, beaten
5 tbsp.	75 mL	butter
½		small onion, chopped
1 or 2		cloves garlic, chopped
4 tbsp.	50 mL	flour
2 cups	500 mL	milk
¾ cup	175 mL	grated Parmesan cheese
3 cups	750 mL	shredded mozzarella cheese
		salt, pepper and nutmeg to taste

Cook the lasagne noodles in plenty of boiling, salted water until tender but not mushy. Drain, then rinse very well with cold water, and set aside.

Rinse the spinach with water, then place in a saucepan, cover, and cook in just the water that clings to the leaves, until wilted—about 5 minutes. Drain thoroughly, pressing out as much excess liquid as possible, then chop coarsely and let cool for a few minutes. Add the ricotta cheese and the eggs and mix well.

Melt 1 tbsp. (15 mL) of the butter in a saucepan over medium heat. Add the chopped onion and garlic and cook until the onion is soft. Remove from heat and add to the spinach mixture.

Melt the remaining 4 tbsp. (50 mL) of butter in the same saucepan. Stir in the flour, cook for a minute or two, then add the milk gradually, stirring constantly to eliminate any lumps. Cook over medium-low heat until the sauce thickens, then add ½ cup (125 mL) of the Parmesan cheese, stir until melted, and remove from heat.

Now you have all the parts. Let's put them together.

Place 4 or 5 of cooked lasagne noodles on the bottom of a greased 9 x 13-inch (22 x 33 cm) baking dish, overlapping the noodles and covering the bottom completely. Over this, spread half of the spinach mixture, and about one-third of the shredded mozzarella. Sprinkle with salt and pepper. Repeat: a layer of noodles, the rest of the spinach mixture, another third of the mozzarella and a sprinkle of salt and pepper. Finally, top with the last layer of noodles, pour on all the cheese sauce, sprinkle with the rest of the mozzarella cheese, and the rest of the Parmesan cheese. Sprinkle the top lightly with nutmeg.

Bake lasagne at 350° F (180° C) for 30 to 35 minutes, until bubbly and lightly browned on top. Let stand at room temperature for at least 10 minutes before serving.

Makes 6 servings.

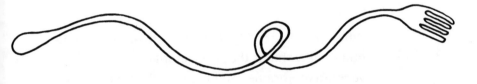

Split Cooking—A Survival Strategy for the Mixed Household

Someone you know and love (or like, anyway) has just turned vegetarian. You fear the worst. Lentils. Brussels sprouts. Rutabaga. Tofu. There will be weird, inconvenient meals of strange foods from foreign countries. You are afraid that making dinner will take five hours. Calm down. It's not as scary as it seems. What you need is a strategy.

- When you dissect a typical meal, you'll usually find quite a few things that a vegetarian *can* eat. The vegetables, for one. And the rice, the salad, the bread. If the main dish is to be, for instance, a steak, this would clearly be your problem area. Easy enough. Just substitute something else—a veggie burger, perhaps (homemade or store-bought), or a vegetable pot pie. Make a lentil loaf or a bean stew or a meatless lasagne—cut it into portions and keep it in the freezer. You'll always have something ready to plunk on a plate instead of the meat.

- If you're making a stir-fry, cook the chicken or beef separately from the vegetables, and toss it together at the end, having reserved a portion to be meatless. You can stir-fry some tofu or beans to add to the vegetarian version of the dish.

- Brown the hamburger for chili or spaghetti sauce separately and add it to the dish after a vegetarian portion has been removed. (Yes, the meat *can* be added later—just simmer it in the sauce for a little while before serving.) Substitute another protein—like crumbled tofu or tempeh or extra beans—to the veggie rendition. In fact, it wouldn't hurt for everyone to double up on the vegetables.

- Keep the fridge stocked with blocks of firm tofu, which easily lends itself to meat-like cooking techniques. Marinate it in barbecue sauce and bake it, bread it and pan-fry it, simmer it in the same sauce you're using to cook the chicken.

- Make a couple of days of the week non-meat for everyone. Experiment with vegetarian versions of familiar dishes—pizza, lasagne, tacos—you may even like them better that way.

- Encourage your resident vegetarian to cook. Have him or her plan the meals and prepare some or all of the dishes. You'll broaden your horizons while splitting the work load. Not a bad plan, on the whole.

Shells Stuffed with Broccoli and Cheese

This is a great buffet dish—easy to serve. Even easier to eat.

24		jumbo pasta shells
1		medium bunch broccoli, coarsely chopped
1 cup	250 mL	ricotta cheese
½ cup	125 mL	shredded Swiss cheese
1		small onion, chopped
2 tbsp.	30 mL	chopped fresh basil
½ tsp.	2 mL	crumbled dried oregano
½ tsp.	2 mL	salt
¼ tsp.	1 mL	pepper
1		(28-oz./796 mL) can diced tomatoes

Cook the jumbo pasta shells in plenty of boiling, salted water until just tender but not falling apart. Drain thoroughly and set aside.

Steam the chopped broccoli until tender but not soft—about 10 minutes. Dump into a mixing bowl and let cool for a few minutes. Add the ricotta cheese, Swiss cheese, onion, basil, oregano and salt and pepper. Toss to combine.

Pour about 1 cup (250 mL) of the diced tomatoes over the bottom of a 9 x 13-inch (22 x 33 cm) baking pan. Mash the tomatoes a bit with a fork to eliminate any big chunks. Now, one at a time, spoon about 1 tbsp. (15 mL) of the cheese mixture into each shell and arrange them, open side up, on top of the tomatoes in the baking dish. After the shells are all filled, pour the remaining tomatoes over and around the shells, and cover the pan with foil. Bake at 375° F (190° C) for 25 to 35 minutes until the shells are heated through and the sauce is bubbly.

Makes about 6 servings.

Stir-fry Crazy

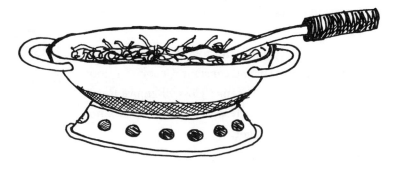

A Basic Stir-fry

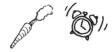

The trick to preparing a panic-free stir-fry is to have all the ingredients cut up and ready to go. If you arrange everything on a platter or tray before you start, this stir-fry should take no more than about 10 minutes to cook. Pick any combination of vegetables from the list on the right, but remember: More is not always better.

1 tbsp.	15 mL	cornstarch
3 tbsp.	45 mL	soy sauce
¾ cup	175 mL	vegetable broth
2 tbsp.	30 mL	vegetable oil
1 tbsp.	15 mL	finely grated fresh ginger root
2		cloves garlic, squished
10 cups	2.5 L	assorted sliced, diced and chopped vegetables (see sidebar)

First, stir together the cornstarch, soy sauce and vegetable broth in a small bowl. Set aside.

Heat the vegetable oil in a wok or very large skillet over high heat. Add the ginger and garlic and cook, stirring, for 15 to 20 seconds. Don't allow the garlic to burn.

Now start tossing the rest of the stuff in. If you're using an onion, throw that into the wok first—it will add flavor to everything. Next, add any *firm* tofu, tempeh or seitan you might be using and let it sizzle a bit. Now, begin adding

Stir-fry inspirations

- Chunked onion
- Chunked green or red pepper, carrots mushrooms, celery
- Broccoli or cauliflower flowerets
- Shredded cabbage, spinach or Chinese greens
- Snow peas
- Bean sprouts
- Green beans or asparagus
- Tofu
- Diced steamed tempeh
- Sliced seitan
- Cashews, peanuts or sesame seeds

vegetables in the order they will take to cook: First the hard vegetables, like carrots. Then things like celery, peppers, broccoli. Then mushrooms and *soft* tofu (if you're using it). And finally add any tender greens, like shredded cabbage, spinach, bok choy or bean sprouts.

As soon as everything is in the wok, pour in the cornstarch mixture and, stirring constantly, cook just until the sauce thickens and becomes glossy. Remove from heat, and serve immediately with hot cooked rice, noodles or whatever you've got.

Makes 3 or 4 servings.

Sprouts

The sprouts that you will most often come across are mung bean and alfalfa. Mung bean sprouts are the ones that are stir-fried in Chinese dishes. They're long and fleshy, with a small bean thing at the top end. They should be crisp, the roots white, and with no slimy or wilted sections. Alfalfa sprouts are usually sold in small plastic boxes. They're thin and delicate, with tiny green leaves at the top. These are usually eaten raw, in salads or on sandwiches. Sometimes you may even come across onion sprouts, broccoli sprouts, radish sprouts or sunflower sprouts. Each one has a distinctive taste—try them all to see what you like.

And as if you didn't already have enough to do, why don't you try sprouting your own sprouts? See page 121 for details.

Spicy Tofu and Eggplant

There's something about the combination of tofu and eggplant that brings out the best in both of them. Feel free to reduce the amount of chili paste if you'd prefer a milder dish—this is very spicy.

1 lb.	500 g	regular tofu, cut into ½-inch (1 cm) cubes
1		medium eggplant, peeled and cut into ½-inch (1 cm) cubes
1 tbsp.	15 mL	soy sauce
1 tsp.	5 mL	brown sugar
2 tsp.	10 mL	sherry
1 tsp.	5 mL	sesame oil
½ tsp.	2 mL	cornstarch
1 tbsp.	15 mL	water
2 tbsp.	30 mL	vegetable oil
1½ tsp.	7 mL	grated fresh ginger root (see page 105)
2		cloves garlic, squished
2 tbsp.	30 mL	Chinese chili paste (see page 76)
2		green onions, chopped

> ### Sesame oil
>
> Used as a seasoning rather than a cooking oil, a little drizzle of sesame oil added to a stir-fry at the last minute provides a lovely sesame flavor. There is no real substitute —simply leave it out if you don't have it. Available in Chinese grocery stores, and some large supermarkets.

While you're preparing all the other ingredients, place the tofu cubes in a colander or strainer set over a bowl to allow the excess water to drain out.

Place the eggplant cubes in a steamer basket over boiling water and steam for about 5 minutes, until soft. Remove from heat. Set aside.

In a small bowl, stir together the soy sauce, brown sugar, sherry, sesame oil, cornstarch and water. Set this aside too.

Okay, now you're ready. Heat the vegetable oil in a wok (or large skillet). Add the ginger and garlic, and stir-fry for just a few seconds. Now add the chili paste, and stir for another, maybe, 30 seconds. Now throw in the tofu cubes, the eggplant, the green onion, and the little dish of soy sauce mixture. Cook, stirring constantly, until the mixture is heated through and thickens slightly.

Serve hot with rice.

Makes 3 or 4 servings.

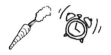

Cashew Noodle Stir-fry

If you can find the thin Chinese noodles that come vacuum packed and precooked, use them in this stir-fry. They add a nice stringy, chewy texture to the dish. Otherwise use any thin pasta—like spaghettini, vermicelli or capellini instead.

12 oz.	350 g	package thin precooked Chinese noodles
		or
8 oz.	250 g	very thin pasta, vermicelli or capellini
1 tbsp.	15 mL	vegetable oil
1 cup	250 mL	cashew pieces
1		medium sweet green or red pepper, thinly sliced
2		stalks celery, sliced
1		(14-oz./398 mL) can baby corn cobs, drained and halved lengthwise
2 cups	500 mL	fresh bean sprouts
4		green onions, slivered
2 tbsp.	15 mL	soy sauce
1 tbsp.	30 mL	Chinese chili paste (or less, or none) (page 76)

If you are using precooked Chinese noodles, open the package and place them in a strainer. Pour boiling water over them and fluff them up with a fork. That's all. They're now ready to use.

If you are using regular pasta, cook it in plenty of boiling water until tender but not mushy, drain thoroughly, and set aside.

Heat the oil in a wok or large skillet. Add cashews, and stir-fry over high heat for 1 minute, until they are lightly golden. Now throw in the sliced green or red pepper, the celery and the baby corn, and stir-fry for about 3 minutes. Add the bean sprouts and the green onions, and cook for just one more minute, until the sprouts are beginning to wilt. Now stir in the noodles, and toss to combine.

In a small bowl, stir together the soy sauce and the chili paste (if you're using it), then add to the noodle mixture, tossing just until heated through. (If you're not using the chili paste, you may want to increase the amount of soy sauce.) Serve immediately.

Makes 4 servings.

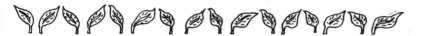

Urban Agriculture
Grow Your Own Bean Sprouts!

Just because you don't live on a 200-acre farm doesn't mean you can't grow your own food. Bean sprouts require no tractor, no giant harvesting machine, no pesticides or herbicides. All you need are some seeds, a jar, a piece of cheesecloth and a dark closet. Interested?

First, buy some mung beans at a bulk food or health food store. (*Never* sprout beans that are meant to be planted outdoors in a garden because they may have been treated with fungicide or other chemicals.) Measure about 1/4 cup (50 mL) mung beans into a 1-quart (1 L) size jar. Any old kind of jar will do—it doesn't even have to have a lid. Fill the jar with cold water and fasten a small square of cheesecloth or other netting over the opening, using a rubber band to hold it in place. Let the beans soak overnight in a dark place (like a closet). In the morning, without removing the cheesecloth, pour off the water, rinse the beans briefly with fresh water, and then drain thoroughly. Now lay the jar down on its side in the dark closet and go away. Repeat the rinsing and draining two or three times a day. You want to keep the beans moist—but they should not be sitting in a puddle.

After a day or two, you'll begin to see small white sprouts appear. Keep rinsing and draining, and in 3 to 5 days, you'll have yourself a crop ready to be harvested. The sprouts can be eaten when they're 1 to 2 inches (2.5 to 5 cm) long.

Yee-haw!

Pad Thai

Pad Thai traditionally contains fish sauce, an ingredient that gives the dish its distinctive flavor. If you avoid all fish and seafood, use soy sauce instead. The taste of the finished dish will be different—but still delicious. Feel free to add other vegetables—snow peas, slivered green pepper, shredded carrot—when you add the bean sprouts and green onion.

8 oz.	250 g	dry rice noodles (or similar amount of regular linguine or spaghetti)
1 tbsp.	15 mL	Thai fish sauce *or* soy sauce
3 tbsp.	45 mL	lime juice
2 tbsp.	30 mL	sugar
1 tbsp.	15 mL	ketchup
½ tsp.	2 mL	crushed hot red pepper flakes
¼ cup	50 mL	vegetable oil
2 cups	500 mL	firm tofu, cut into ¼-inch (1.5 cm) cubes
1 tbsp.	15 mL	chopped garlic
2		eggs, beaten
2 cups	500 mL	bean sprouts
3		green onions, slivered
½ cup	125 mL	ground or finely chopped peanuts
2 tbsp.	30 mL	chopped cilantro (page 27)

If using rice noodles, soak them in warm water for at least 30 minutes or as long as several hours, then drain and set aside. If using regular pasta, cook, then drain, rinse and set aside.

In a small bowl, combine the fish sauce or soy sauce, lime juice, sugar, ketchup and crushed red pepper flakes. Set aside.

Heat the oil in a wok or large skillet. Add the cubed tofu, and fry until golden and beginning to get crisp on all sides. Remove to a bowl, leaving the oil behind.

Add the garlic to the hot oil, cook for 10 seconds, then add the eggs and cook, stirring, until scrambled. Now add the noodles to the wok, mix well, and pour in the fish or soy sauce mixture. Cook, stirring constantly, until the noodles are soft and tender, just a few minutes. You can add up to ¼ cup (50 mL) of water if the mixture seems too dry.

Stir in the bean sprouts, green onions, fried tofu and ground peanuts. Fry for a minute or two. Taste for seasoning, adding more lime or chili if desired. Serve sprinkled with chopped cilantro, additional bean sprouts and a wedge of lime.

Makes 3 to 4 servings.

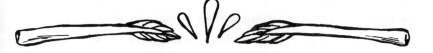

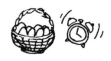

Fried Rice with Vegetables and Seitan or Tempeh

Seitan and tempeh are two of the most meat-like non-meats there are.
You could easily convince someone that they're eating chicken or pork
if you really wanted to. This is a good recipe to experiment with these
two foods.

3 tbsp.	45 mL	vegetable oil
1		egg, slightly beaten
4		whole green onions, sliced
1		clove garlic, squished
1		small carrot, diced
1 cup	250 mL	peas—thawed frozen or cooked fresh
8 oz.	225 g	seitan, cut into 1-inch/2 cm strips
		or
8.5 oz.	240 g	tempeh (approximately 1 package), cut into ½-inch (1 cm) cubes and steamed for 20 minutes
4 cups	1 L	cooked rice—cold leftover rice is perfect
3 tbsp.	45 mL	soy sauce

Heat 1 tbsp./15 mL of the oil in a large skillet or wok, then pour in
the egg and cook, stirring, until scrambled. Remove from the pan and
set aside.

Add the remaining 2 tbsp./30 mL of oil to the pan over high heat.
Add the green onions and garlic and stir-fry for 1 minute. Add the
carrot and peas and continue to stir-fry for 2 more minutes—until
the carrot is just beginning to soften. Add the seitan or tempeh and
heat through, stirring constantly.

Now dump in the rice, soy sauce and the scrambled egg. Stir-fry
until the rice is heated through and the soy sauce is evenly mixed.
Serve immediately.

Makes 2 to 4 servings.

Seitan

Here's a meat alternative that—surprise!—isn't made from soy beans. Instead, seitan is made from wheat gluten—the protein part of wheat—and is a common "mock" meat used in Asian cooking. It can be cut into chunks or slices and, when marinated, has a taste and texture that comes so close to meat that it can make a vegetarian feel guilty. But don't. Seitan is perfectly innocent and totally harmless.

Although seitan isn't as widely available as some of the other meat alternatives, you can often find it in health food stores. It generally comes in vacuum packages, in marinated and plain forms. Seitan is a good source of protein, is very low in fat and has no cholesterol (of course).

Because seitan is such a meat-like thing, it can be thrown, almost undetectably, into a stir-fry, stew or spaghetti sauce. For the intrepid shopper, seitan can sometimes be found in Chinese groceries, in a canned form, masquerading as barbecued duck or pork. Very interesting stuff.

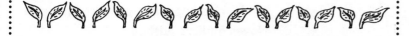

Chilis, Curries, Casseroles and Concoctions

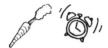 ## Veggie-Packed Chili

This chili is loaded with vegetables, nice and thick, and just spicy enough to make you notice. It's excellent served with Jalapeño Cornbread (page 191). Try folding leftovers into a tortilla, with a dollop of sour cream, for a satisfying lunch.

1		large eggplant, peeled and cut into ½-inch (1 cm) cubes
		or
1 lb.	500 g	firm tofu, frozen, defrosted and crumbled
		or
1 cup	250 mL	texturized vegetable protein granules (TVP)
¼ cup	50 mL	olive or vegetable oil
2		onions, chopped
2		medium zucchini, cut into ½-inch (1 cm) cubes
2		medium red or green peppers, chopped
4		cloves garlic, squished
1		(28-oz./796 mL) can tomatoes, coarsely broken up
3 tbsp.	45 mL	chili powder
1 tbsp.	15 mL	ground cumin
1 tbsp.	15 mL	crumbled dried oregano
1 tsp.	5 mL	pepper

½ tsp.	2 mL	hot pepper flakes (or more, or less)
½ tsp.	2 mL	salt (or to taste)
1		(19-oz./540 mL) can black beans, pinto beans or red kidney beans, drained (or 2 cups/500 mL home-cooked)
1½ cups	375 mL	corn—fresh cut from the cob, or frozen or canned

If you're using the eggplant, place the cubes in a colander set over a bowl, and toss with about 2 tsp. (10 mL) of salt. Let sit for about an hour to drain, then rinse and pat dry with paper towel. This will draw the excess liquid out of the eggplant and help it cook more quickly and reduce any bitterness. If you are in a big hurry, you can skip this step. (If you're using tofu instead, forget we ever mentioned eggplant.) Or, if you're using the TVP, measure the granules into a large bowl and add enough boiling water to cover. Let soak, then drain and, by hand, squeeze out as much of the excess water as possible.

Heat the oil in a large, heavy pot or Dutch oven, and cook the onions, zucchini, peppers and garlic over medium heat for about 5 minutes, until softened. Add either the eggplant cubes, rehydrated TVP or the crumbled tofu (depending on which you're using) and continue to cook, stirring occasionally, for 5 or 10 minutes, until the vegetables are tender. Add the tomatoes with all the juice from the can, the chili powder, cumin, oregano, pepper, hot pepper flakes and salt, and bring the mixture to a boil. Lower the heat and cook gently, stirring once in a while, for about 15 minutes.

Add the beans and the corn to the pot, and cook for another 15 minutes. Taste and adjust the seasoning if necessary.

Serve hot, sprinkled with shredded cheese if you like, over hot cooked rice or with a big chunk of cornbread.

Makes about 8 servings.

Have Your Sweet Potatoes Gone too Far?

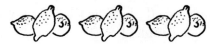

Okay, so you forgot about your sweet potatoes and they are starting to sprout in the bag. Well, all is not lost! You can turn that poor neglected vegetable into a lovely houseplant. Here's how.

Simply poke three toothpicks around the waistline of a sweet potato, and suspend it vertically in a jar of water. Keep it there for a long time. Eventually, if the potato hasn't been treated with some nasty chemical to prevent sprouting, it will begin to grow. First a little sprout, then a longer stem, then it turns into an attractive viney plant. Transfer it to a pot filled with potting soil once it has plenty of roots and a few leaves.

Nifty, isn't it?

Sweet Potato and Pinto Bean Chili

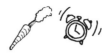

This is an amazing, dirt-cheap, really fast chili. If you don't happen to have pinto beans, use something else—try it with black beans (for that Hallowe'en effect), or good old kidney beans for a more traditional look.

2 tbsp.	30 mL	vegetable oil
2		medium onions, chopped
2 tbsp.	30 mL	Mexican chili powder
1 tsp.	5 mL	ground cumin
1 cup	250 mL	vegetable broth
2		medium sweet potatoes, peeled and cubed
1		(28-oz./796 mL) can diced tomatoes
2		(19-oz./540 mL each) cans pinto (or other) beans, drained and rinsed (or 4 cups/ 1 L home-cooked beans)
1 tsp.	5 mL	salt
1 tsp.	5 mL	crumbled dried oregano
¼ tsp.	1 mL	cayenne (or less, to taste)
½ cup	125 mL	chopped fresh cilantro

Heat the oil in a large saucepan or Dutch oven. Add the onions and cook, stirring, over medium heat until the onions are soft—about 5 minutes. Add the chili powder and the cumin and cook for another minute or so. Add the vegetable broth and the cubed sweet potatoes, reduce the heat to low and cook, covered, until the potatoes are almost tender—about 10 minutes.

Add the tomatoes with all the juice from the can, the beans, salt, oregano and cayenne. Bring to a boil over medium heat, then let simmer until the potatoes are completely tender—about 20 minutes. Remove from heat and stir in the chopped fresh cilantro.

Serve with rice or corn bread and sprinkled with shredded cheese, if you like.

Makes 6 servings.

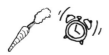 # Cauliflower Curry

This is a fairly mild, but very delicious curry. If you prefer your curry flaming hot, add another fresh hot pepper to the dish when you throw in the peas. Or just sprinkle in some extra cayenne. Serve it with Lentil Dal (page 185), a refreshing Raita (see next page) and Indian Vegetable Pilau (page 151) for an evening in India.

¼ cup	50 mL	vegetable oil
1		medium cauliflower, broken into flowerets
2		medium onions, chopped
¼ cup	50 mL	chopped cilantro
1		small fresh hot pepper, chopped (or ¼ tsp./1 mL cayenne)
1 cup	250 mL	chopped tomato—fresh or canned
1 tsp.	5 mL	ground cumin
½ tsp.	2 mL	ground coriander
½ tsp.	2 mL	turmeric
½ tsp.	2 mL	salt
1		clove garlic, squished
1 cup	250 mL	water

Heat the oil in a (very) large skillet, add the cauliflower pieces and cook over medium heat, until slightly browned, stirring occasionally. This will take 8 to 10 minutes. Remove the cauliflower to a bowl and set aside.

In a blender or food processor, blend together the onions, cilantro, hot pepper, tomatoes, cumin, coriander and turmeric. Pour this mixture into the skillet and cook, stirring, over medium heat until slightly thickened—8 to 10 minutes.

Return the cauliflower to the pan, along with the salt, garlic and water. Cover and cook over medium-low heat for 15 to 20 minutes—until the cauliflower is tender (*not* tender-crisp) and the flavors are nicely blended.

Serve with a cool raita and some rice, or rolled into a tortilla.

Makes 4 to 6 servings.

Two Refreshing Raitas

A spoonful or two of cool and creamy raita is the best way to cool down a hot, spicy curry. Here are two possible variations on this traditional Indian condiment.

Veggie Raita

1½ cups	375 mL	plain yogurt
1		small tomato, finely chopped
1		small cucumber, peeled and finely chopped
1		green onion, chopped
1 tbsp.	15 mL	chopped cilantro
¼ tsp.	2 mL	cumin seeds
		salt and pepper to taste

Fruity Raita

1½ cups	375 mL	plain yogurt
1		banana, peeled and diced
¼ cup	50 mL	grated coconut (unsweetened, preferably)
1 tbsp.	15 mL	chopped fresh mint or cilantro
		salt and pepper, if desired

Combine all the ingredients for whichever raita you're making in a small bowl. Mix well and refrigerate for about 1 hour before serving.

Makes about 2 cups (500 mL).

Potato and Pea Curry

This is the Indian equivalent of an everyday comfort dish. Good old potatoes, it seems, are good old potatoes everywhere. Leftovers are great folded into a tortilla for a quick lunch.

1½ lbs.	750 g	potatoes
2 tbsp.	30 mL	vegetable oil
2 tsp.	10 mL	whole mustard seeds
2		onions, thickly sliced
4		cloves garlic, squished
2 tsp.	10 mL	grated fresh ginger root (page 105)
1 tsp.	5 mL	turmeric
½ tsp.	2 mL	cayenne (or less, or none—if you can't take the heat)
1 tsp.	5 mL	ground cumin
1 tsp.	5 mL	garam masala
½ tsp.	2 mL	salt
½ cup	125 mL	water
1 cup	250 mL	fresh or frozen peas
2 tbsp.	30 mL	chopped fresh mint (if you can get it) or cilantro

Garam Masala

This is an Indian spice mixture that can usually be found in any store that carries a good selection of spices. It usually contains cumin, coriander, cinnamon, cloves and cardamom, and is aromatic, rather than spicy. A reasonable substitute would be a pinch of each of the above.

Peel the potatoes only if they have thick old skins, then cut them up into large cubes (about 1 inch/2.5 cm).

Heat the oil in a large skillet, add the mustard seeds and cook until they start to bounce around in the pan and pop. Lots of fun to watch. Now add the onions, garlic and grated ginger. Cook, stirring, over low heat until soft. Be careful not to burn the garlic and ginger. Add the turmeric, cayenne, cumin, garam masala, salt and the cubed potatoes. Stir around for a minute over medium heat, until the potatoes are coated with the spices. Add the water, lower the heat to a simmer and cook, covered, for 15 to 20 minutes—until the potatoes are tender. Now add the peas and cook, covered, for another 5 minutes. Stir in the mint and serve.

Serve as a side dish with other things, or as a main dish with rice or bread and some yogurt on the side.

Makes 3 or 4 servings.

Chick-Pea Curry

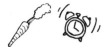

This curry is really mild. But it doesn't have to be. If you want a little heat, add a chopped hot pepper or some cayenne when you add the tomatoes. Leftovers are great stuffed into a pita pocket.

2 tbsp.	30 mL	vegetable oil
1		onion, chopped
1		small piece cinnamon stick
2		cloves garlic, squished
1 tbsp.	15 mL	finely grated fresh ginger root (page 105)
2		tomatoes, chopped (fresh or canned)
2		(19-oz./540 mL) cans chick-peas, drained but reserve the liquid (or 4 cups/1 L home-cooked)
1 tsp.	5 mL	ground cumin
½ tsp.	2 mL	ground coriander
½ tsp.	2 mL	salt

Heat the oil in a large skillet over medium heat. Add the chopped onion and the piece of cinnamon stick, and cook, stirring, until the onion is golden, about 10 minutes. Add the garlic and ginger root, and cook for another 2 or 3 minutes. Dump in the tomatoes and let the mixture simmer for about 10 minutes, until the tomatoes are soft.

Stir in the drained chick-peas, the cumin, coriander and salt. Let this come to a simmer and cook, stirring occasionally, for 10 to 12 minutes, adding up to 1 cup (250 mL) of reserved chick-pea liquid or water to keep the mixture saucy.

Makes about 4 servings.

Eight-Vegetable Stew

Snuggle up to a bowl of this delicious stew on a cold winter evening. It'll make you feel all warm and cozy.

¼ cup	50 mL	olive oil
½ lb.	250 g	small mushrooms, trim stems but leave whole
½ lb.	250 g	whole baby carrots
3		cloves garlic, chopped
1 cup	250 mL	white wine or vegetable broth
¼ lb.	125 g	pearl onions, peeled
2 cups	500 mL	water
2 tbsp.	30 mL	tomato paste
¼ cup	50 mL	chopped fresh parsley
1 tsp.	5 mL	salt
1		large red pepper, cut in strips
1		small zucchini, cut into ½-inch (1 cm) chunks
2 cups	500 mL	broccoli flowerets
1 cup	250 mL	cauliflower flowerets
1		(19-oz./540 mL) can chick-peas, drained (or 2 cups/500 mL home-cooked)

Before you do anything else, prepare all the vegetables and arrange them (artistically) on a platter. This step will most likely take longer than the actual cooking, but it gives you an opportunity to admire all the lovely vegetables before you cook them.

In a large skillet, heat the olive oil over medium heat, and sauté the mushrooms, carrots and garlic for 1 minute. Add the wine or broth and cook over fairly high heat until the liquid is reduced to about ½ cup (125 mL)—about 5 minutes. Don't bother to measure this out, just eyeball it.

Add the onions, water, tomato paste, parsley and salt. Cook, stirring frequently, over high heat until the onions are tender—5 to 7 minutes. Now toss in the red pepper strips, zucchini, broccoli and cauliflower (if you can *bear* to destroy your creation) and cook, stirring, for another 5 to 7 minutes, until all the vegetables are tender but still crisp. Finally, dump in the chick-peas and cook only long enough to heat through.

Serve with rice or mashed potatoes.

Makes 4 servings.

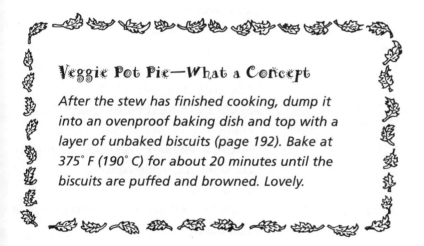

Veggie Pot Pie—What a Concept

After the stew has finished cooking, dump it into an ovenproof baking dish and top with a layer of unbaked biscuits (page 192). Bake at 375° F (190° C) for about 20 minutes until the biscuits are puffed and browned. Lovely.

Spicy Vegetable Couscous

This spicy vegetable concoction can also be served with rice or pasta, if you don't happen to have any couscous in the house.

1 tbsp.	15 mL	vegetable or olive oil
1		small onion, chopped
2		cloves garlic, chopped
1 cup	250 mL	vegetable broth
1 cup	250 mL	peeled butternut squash, cut into ½-inch/1 cm cubes
1		medium zucchini, cut into ½-inch/1 cm cubes
1		(19-oz./540 mL) can chick-peas, drained (2 cups/500 mL home-cooked)
½ tsp.	2 mL	ground cumin
¼ tsp.	1 mL	crushed hot red pepper flakes (or more, if you dare)
½ tsp.	2 mL	curry powder
1		medium tomato, cut into ½-inch/1 cm chunks
¼ cup	50 mL	raisins
		salt and black pepper to taste
1 cup	250 mL	dry couscous
1 cup	250 mL	boiling water

In a large skillet or Dutch oven, heat the oil over medium heat. Add the chopped onion and garlic, and cook until softened, about 5 minutes. Add the vegetable broth and the butternut squash, cover, and let the squash simmer until almost tender—about 15 minutes.

Add the zucchini, chick-peas, cumin, hot pepper flakes and curry powder and stir. Replace the cover and let cook for about 5 minutes. Now add the tomato and raisins, and cook just until heated through. Taste and season with salt and black pepper.

In the meantime, while things are simmering, prepare the couscous. Place the dry couscous into a bowl or saucepan. Pour the boiling water over it, stir, cover and let sit for 10 minutes. Fluff with a fork and scoop into a serving bowl. That's all there is to it.

Spoon the vegetable mixture over the couscous and serve immediately.

Makes 3 to 4 servings.

How to chop an onion without crying

Method 1
Place the onion on a cutting board. Place the cutting board on the front burner of your stove. *Do not turn on the burner!* Now turn on the back burner and chop to your heart's content. The heat (or whatever) will draw the onion fumes away from you, leaving you free to chop tearlessly. Really. (Remember to turn off the back burner when you're done.)

Method 2
Wear contact lenses.

Method 3
Wear a diving mask.

Mushroom Stroganoff with Seitan (or Not)

If you can find seitan in your local health food store and you've never used it, this recipe is the perfect way to give it a try. Seitan (wheat gluten—not scary) has a chewy, meaty texture that goes very nicely with the mushrooms, and adds protein besides. If you're not using the seitan, you can just omit it from the recipe and begin by sautéing the onion and mushrooms.

2 tbsp.	30 mL	vegetable oil
8 oz.	250 g	seitan, cut into ⅛-inch (.25 cm) slices
1 lb.	500 g	mushrooms, cut into quarters
1		onion, chopped
½ cup	125 mL	white wine
1 tbsp.	15 mL	flour
1 cup	250 mL	vegetable broth
¼ cup	50 mL	sour cream
2 tbsp.	30 mL	chopped fresh parsley
		salt and pepper to taste

Heat 1 tbsp. (15 mL) of the oil in a large frying pan, add the seitan slices, and fry over medium heat, turning the slices over as they become slightly crisp and golden. Remove from the pan, leaving as much of the oil behind as possible, and set aside.

Add the remaining 1 tbsp. (15 mL) of oil to the frying pan. Dump in the mushrooms and onion and cook, stirring, over medium heat for 8 to 10 minutes, until the mushrooms have released all their liquid and it has evaporated. Add the wine and cook until it is slightly reduced—about 3 minutes.

Sprinkle the flour over the mushrooms, stir, then pour in the broth and bring the mixture to a boil. Return the seitan slices to the pan, lower the heat and let simmer for a couple of minutes. Add the sour cream and parsley, and season to taste with salt and pepper. Heat through and serve with buttered egg noodles or plain cooked rice.

Makes 2 servings.

Cuban-Style Black Beans

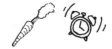

A little Cuban music in the background and—hey!—you're dining in Havana. Well, almost. Try folding leftovers into a tortilla with shredded cheese and lettuce. Delicious.

¼ cup	50 mL	olive oil
1		large onion, chopped
1		large red pepper, chopped
4		cloves garlic, squished
2 tsp.	10 mL	dried, crumbled oregano
2		(19-oz./540 mL) black beans, drained (or 4 cups/1 L cooked black beans)
¾ cup	175 mL	vegetable broth
2 tbsp.	30 mL	vinegar
		salt and pepper to taste

Heat the oil in a large saucepan or Dutch oven over medium heat. Add the onion, red pepper, garlic and oregano, and cook, stirring, until the onions are softened—about 5 minutes. Add about one-quarter of the beans to the pan and mash them with a fork. Pour in the rest of the beans, broth and vinegar and let simmer for about 15 minutes, stirring once in a while. Season to taste with salt and pepper and serve with hot cooked rice.

Makes 4 to 6 servings.

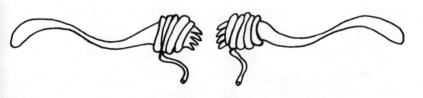

Baked Polenta with Spinach and Cheese

Polenta is a cooked cornmeal dish that may take the place of pasta in an Italian meal. Sometimes it's served on the side (like mashed potatoes), but often polenta is baked into layered casseroles like this one.

10 oz.	284 g	package fresh spinach
1 cup	250 mL	ricotta cheese
¼ cup	50 mL	chopped fresh basil
		salt and pepper to taste
1 recipe		basic polenta (see next page)
2 cups	500 mL	shredded mozzarella cheese

Rummage through the spinach leaves and remove any thick stems or wilted bits. Wash the leaves, then place the wet leaves into a large saucepan and cook, covered, over medium-high heat, stirring occasionally, until the spinach has completely collapsed—about 3 or 4 minutes. Drain well and chop. Set aside.

In a small bowl, mix the ricotta cheese with the basil, salt and pepper. Set this aside too.

Prepare the polenta. While still hot, pour about half of the polenta into a well-greased 9-inch (22 cm)-square baking dish, spreading it out into a smooth layer. Top with the cooked spinach, then the ricotta cheese mixture and sprinkle with half of the shredded mozzarella cheese. Spoon the rest of the polenta on top, and sprinkle with the rest of the mozzarella cheese. Bake at 350° F (180° C) for 35 to 40 minutes, until bubbly and beginning to brown on top.

Makes 4 to 6 servings.

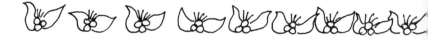

Basic Polenta

Use this recipe to make polenta with spinach and cheese, or top it with a chunky sauce and serve it instead of pasta.

4 cups	1 L	water
1 tsp.	5 mL	salt
1 cup	250 mL	cornmeal
1 tbsp.	15 mL	butter (optional)
¼ cup	50 mL	grated Parmesan cheese (optional)

In a medium-sized heavy pot, bring the water to a boil. Add the salt, then very, very gradually add the cornmeal, stirring like crazy the whole time. The easiest way to do this is to sprinkle the cornmeal from the measuring cup into the water, without ever letting the water stop boiling, and keeping the mixture moving at all times. Clumping is the enemy.

Once you have added all the cornmeal, reduce the heat to low, and continue stirring and simmering for 20 to 30 minutes, or until the mixture is really thick and begins to pull away from the sides of the pan. If you wish to add the butter and Parmesan cheese, stir it in now, and remove from heat. Spoon into a serving dish (quick—before it sets!) and serve hot.

Very Happening Appetizer Recipe

Spread the soft polenta out onto a 9 x 13-inch (22 x 33 cm) baking sheet, and allow to set. Cut into squares or trapezoids, brush with a bit of olive oil, and grill or broil until golden. Serve topped with a dab of goat cheese or pesto, some roasted peppers or whatever. Absolutely now, baby.

Sliceable Polenta

Pour the hot polenta onto a lightly greased baking sheet and chill until firm. These sheets of polenta can now be used in much the same way as lasagne noodles—layered with veggies, sauce and cheese, and baked. You can also spread the soft polenta in a greased pie plate, fill it with something like the filling from Shells Stuffed with Broccoli and Cheese (page 116) or even with pizza toppings, and bake until the filling is done.

Nearly Normal Shepherd's Pie

Really, this is so close to the original that it's almost cheating. But still—for the new vegetarian who is pining for old comfort foods, or for a family meal that is definitely not weird, this is absolutely perfect.

1½ cups	375 mL	TVP (texturized vegetable protein) granules
1½ cups	375 mL	boiling vegetable broth
¼ cup	50 mL	vegetable or olive oil
1		onion, chopped
2		cloves garlic, squished
1		sweet red or green pepper, diced
1		medium carrot, diced
2 cups	500 mL	sliced fresh mushrooms
1 cup	250 mL	fresh or frozen peas or corn kernels
1 cup	250 mL	ketchup, spaghetti sauce, salsa (or a mixture)
4		medium potatoes, peeled and cut into chunks
2 tbsp.	30 mL	butter (or non-dairy margarine)
½ cup	125 mL	milk (or soy milk)
		salt and pepper to taste
		pinch of paprika

In a bowl, combine the TVP granules with the vegetable broth, and soak.

Meanwhile, heat the oil in a large skillet. Add the onion and garlic and cook over medium heat for a couple of minutes—until softened. Add the peppers, carrot and mushrooms and cook for 5 to 7 minutes, until the carrots are almost tender.

Add the rehydrated TVP to the skillet and cook, stirring occasionally and scraping up the bottom of the skillet, for about 5 minutes. Add the peas or corn, and the ketchup (or whatever), and cook for 8 to 10 minutes, stirring once in a while. If the mixture seems too thick, you can add another ½ cup (125 mL) broth or water as it cooks. Season to taste with salt and pepper and dump into a 9-inch (22 cm) square baking dish (or ovenproof casserole of similar size).

In the meantime, make the mashed potatoes. Cook or steam the diced potatoes until quite soft. Drain thoroughly, then mash until smooth with the butter and milk. Season with salt and pepper, and spread while still warm over the vegetable mixture in the baking dish. (A sprinkle of paprika on top is a cheery touch.)

Bake at 350° F (180° C) for 30 to 40 minutes, until the top is golden and the veggie mixture is heated through and bubbling.

Makes 4 to 6 servings.

Texturized Vegetable Protein (TVP)

Texturized vegetable protein (also known as texturized soy protein) is made by processing soy flour in such a way as to turn it into chewy little pellets or chunks which can be added to other foods in place of meat, or as a meat extender. The granular form of TVP is great in chili or spaghetti sauce, and the larger chunky kind can be used in place of beef or chicken in stews. TVP is available in a dehydrated form which must be soaked in boiling water (or vegetable stock) before it can be added to your recipe.

TVP contains about 70 percent protein and retains most of the bean's dietary fiber. It can be found in natural or bulk food stores and may have different brand names, depending on the manufacturer. In its dry form, TVP can be stored at room temperature (like cereal).

Using TVP in place of ground beef in a portion of the recipe makes it easy to accommodate both vegetarians and non-vegetarians in one fell swoop, and to provide a protein alternative in a familiar dish.

Vegetarian Moussaka

Moussaka is the perfect dish to serve when you're entertaining your carnivorous friends or family. Who could care that there's no meat when they're eating something so good? Singing, dancing and plate-smashing after dinner are optional (but fun). This goes nicely with Authentic Greek Salad (page 66) and Spanakopita (page 148).

2		eggplants
2 tbsp.	30 mL	olive oil
1 cup	250 mL	crumbled feta cheese

Custard

2 tbsp.	30 mL	butter
2 tbsp.	30 mL	flour
¾ cup	175 mL	milk
1 tsp.	5 mL	salt
		nutmeg and pepper
2		eggs
1 cup	250 mL	ricotta cheese

Sauce

2		medium onions, chopped
1		medium zucchini, diced
½		medium red or green pepper, diced
2		cloves garlic, chopped
2 tbsp.	15 mL	olive oil
1 tsp.	5 mL	crumbled oregano
¼ tsp.	1 mL	cinnamon
		salt and pepper
2 cups	500 mL	diced tomatoes, fresh or canned
3 tbsp.	45 mL	tomato paste

Without peeling them, slice the eggplants into ½-inch (1 cm) thick slices and salt on both sides. Stand them upright (as much as possible) in a colander and allow the liquid to drain for about 30 minutes or so. (This step helps remove the excess water from the eggplant and reduces any bitterness.) Rinse with water, and pat dry. In batches, brush the eggplant slices with the olive oil and broil in a single layer on a baking sheet until lightly browned (about 2 minutes per side), turning them once. Set aside.

Meanwhile, don't just stand there—make the custard. In a saucepan, melt the butter over medium heat. Stir in the flour and cook for a couple of minutes. Stir in the milk, and cook until smooth and thickened. Remove from heat and stir in the salt, some nutmeg and pepper, the eggs and ricotta. Set this aside too.

Now, make the tomato sauce. In a skillet, cook the chopped onions, zucchini, pepper and garlic with the olive oil until softened. Stir in the oregano, cinnamon, salt and pepper, and cook for a minute or so. Add the tomatoes and tomato paste, and simmer the sauce for about 10 minutes, until slightly thickened.

Okay—now put it all together. Spread half of the tomato sauce in a deep casserole dish, and top with half of the eggplant. Sprinkle with half of the feta cheese, then spread on the rest of the tomato sauce. Layer on the rest of the eggplant, top this with all of the custard, and sprinkle on the rest of the feta cheese.

Bake at 350° F (180° C) for 50 minutes to 1 hour, until the top is browned and set. Let it stand for about 15 minutes before trying to cut into squares.

Makes 4 to 6 (generous) servings.

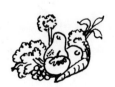

Incredible Onion Tart

You might not believe that a tart filled with nothing but, well, onions could really be this good. But it is. Incredible, isn't it?

1 cup	250 mL	biscuit mix, homemade (page 192) or a commercial brand
1 tsp.	5 mL	crumbled, dried sage
⅓ cup	75 mL	milk
¼ cup	50 mL	butter
4		large onions, thinly sliced
1		egg
½ cup	125 mL	milk
½ tsp.	2 mL	salt
		pepper to taste

In a medium bowl, stir together the biscuit mix, sage and milk. Squish the dough into the bottom and up the sides of an 8-inch (20 cm) pie plate. Set aside.

Melt the butter in a large skillet over medium heat. Add the sliced onion and cook, stirring occasionally, for 12 to 15 minutes, until the onion slices are golden brown. Let cool slightly, then dump into the biscuit-lined pie plate.

In a small bowl, beat together the egg, milk, salt and pepper. Pour over the onion slices. Bake at 400° F (200° C) for 20 to 25 minutes, until the top is lightly browned and the pie is set.

Makes 4 servings.

Oven-Roasted Carrot and Sweet Potato Casserole

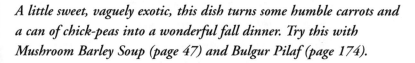

A little sweet, vaguely exotic, this dish turns some humble carrots and a can of chick-peas into a wonderful fall dinner. Try this with Mushroom Barley Soup (page 47) and Bulgur Pilaf (page 174).

4		onions, sliced
2 tbsp.	30 mL	vegetable oil
1		(19-oz./540 mL) can chick-peas, drained (2 cups/500 mL home-cooked)
4		large carrots, cut into ½-inch/1 cm chunks
2 or 3		large sweet potatoes, peeled and cut into ½-inch/1 cm chunks
¼ cup	50 mL	raisins
¼ cup	50 mL	sugar
½ tsp.	2 mL	cinnamon
2 tbsp.	30 mL	vegetable broth

In a large skillet, sauté the onions in 2 tbsp./30 mL of the oil until soft and golden. Spread evenly in a 9 x 13-inch (22 x 33 cm) baking dish. Sprinkle the chick-peas over the onions.

In a large bowl, toss together the carrots, sweet potatoes, raisins, sugar, cinnamon and the vegetable broth. Dump this over the chick-peas, and spread out evenly to cover everything. Bake at 400° F (200° C) for 35 to 45 minutes, basting the top occasionally with some of the liquid from the bottom of the baking dish, until the vegetables are tender and browned.

Makes 6 to 8 servings.

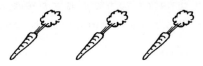

Spanakopita

The phyllo crust makes this dish seem like a lot of work (not true). It tastes as delicious as it looks.

1 lb.	500 g	fresh spinach
1 cup	250 mL	butter
1		medium onion, chopped
½ lb.	250 g	feta cheese, crumbled
2 cups	500 mL	ricotta cheese (one 500 g container)
4		eggs, slightly beaten
1 tsp.	5 mL	salt
¼ tsp.	1 mL	pepper
12		*full sheets* phyllo pastry, defrosted

Rinse the spinach and trim off any big tough stems. Cook it in a large pot, adding no additional water, until wilted—about 5 minutes. Place in a colander and squeeze out the excess liquid. Chop coarsely and set aside.

Melt 1 tbsp. (15 mL) of the butter in a skillet, and cook the chopped onion until soft. Add the chopped spinach and sauté for a couple of minutes. Let cool slightly, then add the feta, ricotta and the beaten eggs. Mix well.

Phyllo Pastry—It's Not as Scary as You Think

Working with phyllo pastry isn't hard, as long as you remember to treat it with a little tender loving care. Take the package of frozen phyllo pastry out of the freezer the day before you want to use it, and place it in the refrigerator to defrost. If you have forgotten to do this, don't try to defrost it at room temperature (or, worse, in the microwave). Just don't. Really. When you are ready to use it, open the box and remove the sleeve containing the pastry. Unwrap it carefully, then unfold the pastry leaves onto a dish towel. Work quickly, keeping the pastry covered with another dish towel to prevent it from drying out. When you are finished, re-roll the pastry, slide it back into the plastic sleeve, seal it tightly and put it back into the freezer. Phyllo pastry can be safely refrozen.

Melt the rest of the butter in a small saucepan.

Meanwhile, unroll the phyllo pastry (see note) and remove 12 full sheets of phyllo. Set them aside, covered with a dish towel. Immediately (quick, before you forget!) roll up the rest of the pastry and return it to the package.

With a pastry brush, brush a 9 x 13-inch (22 x 33 cm) baking dish generously with melted butter. Lay one sheet of phyllo on the bottom of the dish, letting the extra climb up the sides of the baking dish. Brush this sheet with butter and lay another one on top. Repeat this procedure, until you have lined the bottom of the pan with *6 layers* of phyllo, each one brushed with butter. Spread the spinach filling over this. Now cover the filling with a sheet of phyllo, letting the excess overhang the sides of the dish. Brush it with butter, add another sheet, brush with butter (etc., etc.) until you've used up all the rest of the phyllo—making *6 layers* on top. Very gently, using a rubber spatula, tuck the excess overhanging pastry down along the sides of the baking dish—as if you were tucking sheets under a mattress. Brush the top thoroughly with butter. There may be butter left over—save it for another use.

Bake at 350° F (180° C) for 45 minutes, until the top is golden and slightly puffed.

An Appetizing Idea!

Use this same recipe to make little hors d'oeuvres-sized spanakopita triangles. Here's how:

Cut each sheet of phyllo pastry into 4 lengthwise strips. Brush each strip with some melted butter, then place a tablespoon (15 mL) of the filling at one end. Now, fold it into triangles following the diagram. Place on a greased baking sheet, brush tops with butter, and bake at 350° F (180° C) for 15 to 20 minutes, until golden brown and crisp.

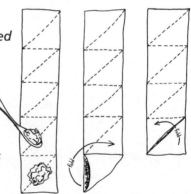

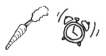

Spicy Beans and Rice

If you want to make this dish with brown rice, increase the amount of vegetable broth to 3 cups (750 mL). And while you're at it, use black beans or pinto beans or even a can of mixed beans instead of the red kidney beans. It's your baby now.

2 tbsp.	30 mL	vegetable or olive oil
1		onion, chopped
1		medium green pepper, chopped
1		stalk celery, finely chopped
2		cloves garlic, squished
½ tsp.	2 mL	crumbled dried oregano
½ tsp.	2 mL	crumbled dried thyme
½ tsp.	2 mL	cayenne (or less—*this is spicy*)
2 cups	500 mL	vegetable broth
2 tbsp.	30 mL	tomato paste
1 cup	250 mL	white rice
1		(19-oz./540 mL) can red kidney beans, drained
½ tsp.	2 mL	salt

Heat the vegetable oil in a large saucepan. Add the chopped onion, green pepper, celery and garlic and cook, stirring, over medium-low heat until the vegetables begin to soften—8 to 10 minutes. Stir in the oregano, thyme and cayenne.

Stir in the vegetable broth and tomato paste, then add the rice, beans and salt and bring to a boil. Lower the heat to a simmer, cover the saucepan, and let cook until the rice is tender and the liquid is absorbed—20 to 25 minutes. Brown rice will take 5 to 10 minutes longer to cook.

Serve immediately.

Makes about 4 servings.

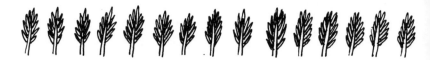

Indian Vegetable Pilau

Make this rice dish the centerpiece of a wonderful Indian feast—with some Chick-Pea Curry (page 133), a yogurt Raita (page 131), and an assortment of store-bought chutneys.

5 tbsp.	75 mL	butter (or non-dairy margarine)
2		onions, chopped
½ tsp.	2 mL	cinnamon
1 tsp.	5 mL	grated fresh ginger root
4 cups	1 L	mixed diced fresh vegetables—potato, sweet potato, peas, carrots, green or red pepper, cauliflower, green beans, zucchini, cooked chick-peas, whatever
2 ½ cups	625 mL	raw basmati rice (or any long-grain rice)
1 tsp.	5 mL	turmeric
4 cups	1 L	water
1 tsp.	5 mL	salt
½ cup	125 mL	raisins

Heat the butter in a large pot and cook the onions until they are golden. Add the cinnamon and ginger, stir, then add all the vegetables, the rice and the turmeric. Cook this business over medium heat for about 5 minutes, stirring frequently. Add the water and salt, and bring to a boil. Turn the heat down very low, cover the pot with a tight-fitting lid, and cook for 20 to 25 minutes, until all the water is absorbed.

Fluff the pilau with a fork, and add the raisins. Dump it into a greased casserole and bake, covered, at 350° F (180° C) for about 20 minutes.

Makes about 8 servings.

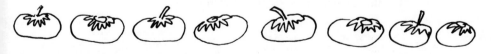

Deeply Personal Pizzas

 ## Pizza with Tomato Sauce and Whatever

Old pizza-maker's trick for making tomato and cheese pizzas: sauce first, then cheese, then the veggies on top of the cheese. This allows the steam from the vegetables to escape, and prevents sogginess. Try it for yourself.

1		12-inch (30 cm) unbaked pizza crust or ½ recipe all-purpose yeast dough (page 187)
1 cup	250 mL	spaghetti sauce—homemade (page 95) or a good quality commercial sauce
2 cups	500 mL	shredded mozzarella cheese toppings (see next page, if you need inspiration)

Spread the spaghetti sauce evenly over the unbaked pizza crust in the baking pan (an official pizza pan, if you have one, or a cookie sheet). Sprinkle with the shredded mozzarella cheese, then top with whatever toppings you want to use. Bake at 425° F (220° C) for about 25 minutes, until the crust is browned when you peek underneath.

Makes one 12-inch (30 cm) pizza—3 to 4 servings. Or less.

Clever idea: Use the entire batch of dough and make 2 pizzas at once. Bake one and stash the second one in the freezer for a sudden midnight snack. You'll be soooo glad you did.

Pizza Topping Ideas (some obvious, some not so obvious)

- Fresh mushrooms
- Green or red peppers
- Onions
- Plum tomatoes
- Grilled eggplant
- Sun-dried tomatoes
- Broccoli
- Roasted red peppers
- Hot pepper rings
- Marinated artichoke hearts
- Green or black olives
- Corn niblets
- Thinly sliced potato
- Pineapple chunks (eeech, personally)

Roasted Red Peppers (You won't be sorry you did this.)

When red peppers are in season, and you can buy beautiful ones quite cheaply, make a big batch of roasted red peppers to freeze. You may not feel like it right now, but in February when red peppers cost as much as a month's rent, you'll be so happy to have these stashed away.

Cut the peppers in half lengthwise through the stem end, and remove the seeds and the spongy stuff inside. If you have a barbecue, place peppers, skin side down on the grill and roast them until the skin turns black. Totally.

If you don't have access to a barbecue, just arrange seeded pepper halves, skin side up on a baking sheet in the oven, and broil close to the element until black.

When your peppers are well-charred, toss them into a covered container or a plastic bag and let them steam for a few minutes, until they are cool enough to handle. Now completely peel away the blackened skin, and place the peppers on a cookie sheet. Put the cookie sheet in the freezer and let the peppers freeze solid, then remove from the cookie sheet, pack them into plastic bags and put them back into the freezer.

Congratulations. You are now the proud owner of a whole bunch of individually frozen roasted red peppers. They can be chopped and tossed with cooked pasta or rice, slivered into a salad or layered on a sandwich.

Pizza with Pesto, Goat Cheese and Sun-Dried Tomatoes

Use either homemade or store-bought pesto sauce to make this deliciously different pizza. You may never go back to tomato sauce again.

1 cup	250 mL	pesto sauce, homemade (page 97) or store-bought
1		12-inch (30 cm) unbaked pizza crust or ½ recipe all-purpose yeast dough (page 187)
½ cup	125 mL	sun-dried tomatoes (packed in oil) cut into strips
5 oz.	140 g	goat cheese (with or without herbs)

Spread the pesto sauce evenly over the unbaked pizza crust in the baking pan (an official pizza pan, if you have one, or a cookie sheet). Sprinkle with the sun-dried tomato strips, and top with crumbled goat cheese. Bake at 425° F (220° C) for about 25 minutes, until the crust is browned when you peek underneath.

Makes one 12-inch (30 cm) pizza—3 to 4 servings. Or less.

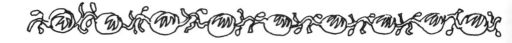

Pizza with Sweet and Sour Caramelized Onions

This may sound like a very strange pizza, but it is absolutely, incredibly amazing. And everyone will think you are a brilliant cook.

2 tbsp.	30 mL	olive oil
1 tbsp.	15 mL	butter
3		onions, thinly sliced
3 tbsp.	45 mL	balsamic vinegar
1 tbsp.	15 mL	sugar
½ tsp.	2 mL	salt
5 oz.	140 g	goat cheese (with or without herbs)
1		12-inch (30 cm) unbaked pizza crust or ½ recipe all-purpose yeast dough (page 187)
¼ cup	50 mL	pine nuts

First, make the caramelized onions. Heat the olive oil and butter in a large skillet over medium-low heat. Add the sliced onions and cook, stirring occasionally, until deep golden brown—about 30 minutes— over fairly low heat. Add the balsamic vinegar, sugar and salt and cook for 5 minutes, until the liquid has almost completely evaporated.

Next, smoosh the goat cheese as evenly as possible over the unbaked crust in the baking pan (an official pizza pan, if you have one, or a cookie sheet). Spread the onions over this, then sprinkle with the pine nuts. Bake at 425° F (220° C) for about 25 minutes, until the crust is browned when you peek underneath.

Makes 1 serving. Just kidding. Maybe 2 or 3.

Random Delights

Baked Barbecue Tofu Steaks

This is a tofu recipe for people who don't think they like tofu. The extra firm tofu holds up nicely when baked with sauce and has a texture that appeals to the newly vegetarianized.

1 pkg.	300 g	extra-firm tofu
1 cup	250 mL	barbecue sauce—any kind you like (try honey garlic or teriyaki)

Cut tofu into ½-inch (1 cm) thick slices and place in a bowl. Pour in the barbecue sauce, turning the slices so that they are coated on all sides. Cover bowl and marinate, refrigerated, for at least 1 hour—but overnight is even better.

Dump the entire contents of the bowl—tofu, sauce and all—into a baking dish big enough to arrange the slices in a single layer. Bake at 375° F (190° C) for about 30 minutes, turning the slices over a couple of times and basting with the sauce.

Serve hot, with some rice or potatoes to soak up the sauce.

Makes 2 or 3 servings.

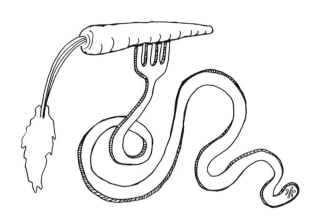

Breaded Tofu Fingers

Vegetarian fish sticks, really. Great kid food. Don't forget the dipping sauce.

1 pkg.	300 g	extra-firm tofu
½ cup	125 mL	dry bread crumbs
¼ tsp.	1 mL	salt
¼ tsp.	1 mL	pepper
¼ tsp.	1 mL	crumbled oregano
¼ tsp.	1 mL	garlic powder
¼ cup	50 mL	flour
1		egg, beaten

Cut the block of tofu into fingers—about ½-inch (1 cm) thick and 3-inches (8 cm) long. More or less.

In a small bowl, combine the bread crumbs, salt, pepper, oregano and garlic powder. Measure flour into another small bowl. Have the egg ready in a third bowl.

Now. First toss the tofu fingers in the flour, then dip each one into the beaten egg, and roll it in the bread crumb mixture. (The flour step, by the way, helps bind the egg and crumbs to the tofu, so that the crumbs don't just fall off.) Place the breaded fingers on a well-greased cookie sheet and bake at 375° F (190° C) for about 30 minutes, turning them over halfway through.

Serve the fingers hot with dipping sauces—ketchup, sweet and sour sauce, plum sauce, barbecue sauce, hot mustard, whatever.

Makes about 16 fingers.

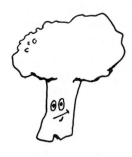

Unexpectedly Delicious Lima Loaf

This is exactly what your friends were worried about, isn't it? Lima beans. And in a loaf, yet. Well, surprise! This dish is so delicious your lima-phobic friends will be begging for a taste, and leftovers make a great sandwich with lettuce, tomato and onion.

1		(19-oz./540 mL) can lima beans, drained (or 2 cups/500 mL home-cooked)
1 cup	250 mL	bread crumbs (seasoned ones are nice here)
½		medium sweet green or red pepper, finely chopped
½		medium onion, finely chopped
¼ cup	50 mL	chopped cashews or almonds
2		eggs
½ cup	125 mL	milk
2 tbsp.	30 mL	butter, melted (plus more for basting) salt and pepper to taste

In a large bowl, mash the lima beans with a fork or potato masher until they are broken up but not puréed. Add the bread crumbs, green or red pepper, onion, cashews, eggs, milk and 2 tbsp. (30 mL) of melted butter. Stir until well mixed, and season to taste with salt and pepper.

Turn this mixture into a very well-greased loaf pan and bake at 350° F (180° C) for 1 hour, basting the top with melted butter every 15 minutes or so. The loaf should be lightly browned on top and puffed, and a knife inserted into the middle should come out fairly clean. Run a knife around the sides of the pan to loosen the loaf, then turn out onto a plate to serve.

Makes 4 to 6 servings.

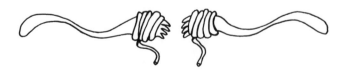

Don't You Just Hate it When That Happens?

You've killed yourself making a delicious loaf (like this one) and, when you try to remove it from the pan, only half of it comes out. Rats. Well, next time here's what you can do to prevent your loaf from sticking: Grease the pan, then line the bottom with a piece of waxed paper, cut to fit, and grease the waxed paper. Bake as usual. Loosen the sides and the loaf will plop right out.

Stuffed Portobello Mushrooms

Portobello mushrooms are, basically, the steak of the vegetable world. Serve one of these per person as a side dish or light main dish, or two per person for a hearty dinner.

4		medium portobello mushrooms
1 tbsp.	15 mL	olive or vegetable oil
1		medium carrot, finely diced
1		medium onion, finely chopped
½		sweet green pepper, finely chopped
1		clove garlic, squished
1 cup	250 mL	cooked brown rice
1 tbsp.	15 mL	chopped fresh basil (or 1 tsp./5 mL dried)
1 tsp.	5 mL	crumbled dried oregano
		salt and pepper to taste
		olive oil for drizzling
		grated Parmesan cheese for sprinkling (optional)

Wipe the mushrooms carefully with a paper towel and remove the stems. Set the caps aside, and chop the stems finely.

Heat the oil in a large skillet over medium heat. Add the chopped mushroom stems, the carrot, onion, green pepper and garlic. Cook, stirring, until the vegetables are softened—8 to 10 minutes. Remove from heat and stir in the rice, basil and oregano. Season to taste with salt and pepper.

Arrange the mushrooms, gill side up, in a lightly greased baking dish. Fill caps with the rice mixture, dividing it equally among the mushrooms, packing it down lightly. Drizzle the tops with a bit more olive oil and a sprinkle of Parmesan cheese (if desired). Bake at 400° F (200° C) for 20 to 30 minutes, until the mushrooms are tender and the filling is heated through.

Makes 2 to 4 servings.

Other Stuffing Suggestions

- Vary this recipe by adding chopped spinach or shredded zucchini to the pan with the onions and carrots.
- Try stuffing big portobello mushrooms with the same mixture your Aunt Gertrude uses in her Thanksgiving turkey.
- Instead of the brown rice in this recipe, try cooked orzo or any small pasta.

Yikes! I didn't know there was meat in there!

Beneath the seemingly vegetarian façade of many commercial food products lurks meat, fish and other non-vegetarian ingredients. These can be in the form of animal fat (like lard or tallow), meat extracts or broth (like chicken or beef in vegetable soups), or even fish. The only way to be sure you're not eating this stuff is to become an obsessive label-reader. Here are a few surprises you might never have considered:

- Packaged crackers (even plain ones) may be made with animal fat (lard or tallow).

- Worcestershire sauce contains anchovies (okay, so that's a fish—but still).

- Some brands of cookies are made with lard (pork fat) or tallow (beef fat).

- Vegetable lasagne sometimes contains chicken broth.

- Canned chili-style beans contain lard.

- Fruit-flavored jelly powder is made with gelatin—an animal extract.

- Many brands of yogurt contain gelatin.

- Some bottled stir-fry sauces contain oyster sauce which is, yes, made from oysters.

- Even a non-meat kind of commercial spaghetti sauce may contain beef or chicken extract or broth.

- Canned vegetable soup will probably contain chicken or beef extract unless it specifically says "vegetarian" on the label.

Barbecued Portobello Burgers

Thick, juicy, meaty. These mushrooms were born to be grilled. For a perfect summer meal, serve this with Crepes Filled with Ratatouille (page 92) and Corn and Tomato Salad (page 61).

4		large portobello mushroom caps
½ cup	125 mL	olive oil
¼ cup	50 mL	balsamic vinegar
2 tbsp.	30 mL	chopped fresh parsley
2		cloves garlic, squished
½ tsp.	2 mL	salt
½ tsp.	2 mL	pepper

Wipe mushrooms with a paper towel or dry cloth and remove stems (save these for your stock bag—page 40). Place tops in a clean zip-top plastic bag.

Combine the olive oil, balsamic vinegar, parsley, garlic, salt and pepper in a small bowl. Pour into the bag with the mushroom caps. Using a drinking straw, suck out as much of the air from the bag as possible, and zip the top shut. Let the mushrooms marinate, refrigerated, for 4 to 6 hours.

To cook, remove the mushroom caps from the bag and place them on a preheated barbecue grill, with the gill side down. Grill until the caps begin to soften, basting occasionally with the marinade, then turn the caps over and grill cap side down until heated through and soft.

Remove carefully from the barbecue, taking care not to lose any of the delicious juice, and place each cap on a fresh hamburger bun. Top with whatever you like (sliced onions, tomatoes, hot peppers, shredded mozzarella, lettuce, you know) and eat. If you can stand to have everyone watching you, that is. Go ahead, share. Isn't that why you made extra?

Makes 4 servings.

Fabulous Side Dish Idea!

Grill these portobello mushrooms and, instead of serving them on a bun, slice them crosswise about ¼-inch (.5 cm) thick and serve, drizzled with a little additional olive oil and balsamic vinegar, as a side dish or an appetizer. Who wouldn't love this?

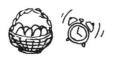

Grillable Tofu Veggie Burgers

Make a batch of these burgers and freeze them on a baking sheet lined with waxed paper. They're better (and cheaper) than store-bought veggie burgers and will make you the envy of even the most committed carnivore at the next barbecue.

1 lb.	454 g	firm tofu, frozen and thawed
¼ cup	50 mL	olive or vegetable oil
1		onion, chopped
½ lb.	250 g	mushrooms, chopped
1		medium carrot, grated
1½ cups	375 mL	cooked brown or white rice
1½ cups	375 mL	bread crumbs
½ cup	125 mL	barbecue sauce—any kind (a smoky kind is nice)
2 tbsp.	30 mL	cornstarch
1 tsp.	5 mL	salt
¼ tsp.	1 mL	pepper
1 cup	250 L	frozen peas or corn (or some of each), thawed
2		eggs

By hand, squeeze as much of the water out of the thawed tofu as possible, and crumble it finely into a large bowl.

Heat the oil in a medium skillet, add the chopped onion and mushrooms, and cook until all the liquid has evaporated and the mixture is beginning to brown slightly. This will take 8 to 10 minutes. Add to the crumbled tofu in the bowl.

Add the grated carrot, rice, bread crumbs, barbecue sauce, cornstarch, salt and pepper. Mix gently. Now put the thawed peas or corn (or both) into the container of a blender or food processor with the eggs. Whirl until the eggs are beaten and the corn and peas are chopped. Add to the mixture in the bowl, and stir until everything is well combined.

Wet your hands and form the burger mixture into patties, using about ½ cup (125 mL) for each patty. Flatten them into a seriously burger shape, and place on a waxed-paper-lined plate. You should end up with about 8 burgers.

To grill your Tofu Veggie Burgers, brush each one with a bit of vegetable or olive oil on both sides and place on a preheated grill over medium heat. Cook until the bottom has begun to brown, then *very* carefully turn them over and grill the other side. If you want, you can brush the cooked side with a bit of barbecue sauce as it continues to cook. Serve in a fresh hamburger bun with lots of the usual stuff.

To bake your Tofu Veggie Burgers, place on a well-oiled cookie sheet and bake at 375° F (190° C) for about 30 minutes, turning them over halfway through. Serve as above.

Or, finally, you can simply pan-fry them in a bit of vegetable oil, turning them over to cook both sides. And ditto on the serving suggestions.

Makes about 8 burgers.

Teriyaki Tempeh Kabobs

This looks enough like meat to make a vegetarian feel, well, uncomfortable. Relax, it's just soy beans.

1 package		(8.5 oz./240 g) tempeh
⅓ cup	75 mL	soy sauce
2 tbsp.	30 mL	brown sugar
2 tbsp.	30 mL	vinegar or lemon juice
1 tbsp.	15 mL	vegetable oil
2		cloves garlic, squished
1 tsp.	5 mL	finely grated fresh ginger root
4		bamboo skewers soaked in hot water for 30 minutes

Cut the block of tempeh into ½-inch (1 cm) cubes. Place in a steamer over boiling water, and steam for 20 minutes. Remove to a bowl.

Meanwhile, mix together the soy sauce, brown sugar, vinegar or lemon juice, oil, garlic and ginger. Pour this mixture over the tempeh and stir to coat the cubes evenly. Let marinate for at least 2 hours (or overnight).

Skewer the tempeh cubes onto the bamboo skewers, leaving a little space between the cubes so that they cook evenly. Grill, turning often and basting with the marinade, on a preheated barbecue. Or place on a baking sheet and broil in the oven, basting with marinade and turning to cook all sides.

Serve hot as a main dish or appetizer.

Makes 4 servings as a main dish.

Tempeh

Tempeh is unusual stuff, there's no doubt about it. A traditional Indonesian food, tempeh is made from soybeans that have been partially cooked, mixed with a culture (think *yeast* or *yogurt*), then pressed into slabs and allowed to ferment. After a period of time, the tempeh is frozen to stop the fermentation. Tempeh is, therefore, most commonly sold as a frozen product.

As a result of this rather complicated process, tempeh develops an interesting, mushroom-like flavor, chewy texture and becomes highly digestible. After an initial steaming, tempeh can be diced and thrown into a stir-fry, baked or grilled with barbecue sauce, or just chopped up, mixed with stuff, and eaten as a salad or sandwich filling. It is an excellent source of protein, is high in fiber and contains both calcium and B vitamins.

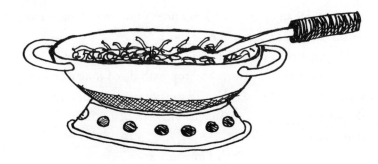

Full Meal Burritos

This is no small snack. This is a fully loaded, knife-and-fork burrito that will make you very happy.

3 tbsp.	45 mL	olive or vegetable oil
3		green onions, finely chopped
4		cloves garlic, squished
1		sweet red or green pepper, chopped
1 or 2		fresh hot peppers, minced
10 oz.	284 g	package fresh spinach, chopped
2		(19-oz./540 mL) cans black beans, drained (or 4 cups/1 L home-cooked)
		salt and pepper to taste
4		large flour tortillas, warmed
2 cups	500 mL	cooked white rice or Mexican red rice (page 173)
2		tomatoes, diced
2 cups	500 mL	shredded Monterey Jack cheese
		salsa and sour cream on the side

Heat the oil in a large skillet over medium heat. Add the onions, garlic, sweet pepper and hot peppers, and cook, stirring, until the onions begin to soften—8 to 10 minutes. Add the spinach and continue to cook until the spinach is wilted, then add the black beans. Cook, stirring occasionally, for about 5 minutes, until everything is combined. Season to taste with salt and pepper.

Place a tortilla on a plate, add a spoonful of cooked rice, a big scoop of the bean mixture, and top with diced tomatoes and sprinkle with shredded cheese. Fold over the bottom and top, then roll in the sides and place, seam side down, on a plate. Serve with salsa and sour cream.

Don't even try eating this in your car.

Makes 4 large burritos.

7. Sidekicks

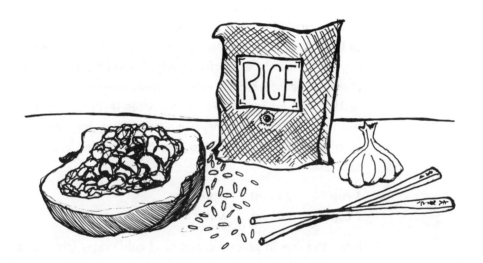

Good Old Grains

Rice-Cooking Basics

Rice is your friend. As a vegetarian, you're bound to run into it a lot, so you may as well learn to cook it well. Lucky for you, this is easy to do.

White Rice

Nothing is simple. All white rice is not the same. There are long-grain, short-grain and medium-grain varieties of white rice. There is Indian basmati rice, Thai jasmine rice and Italian arborio rice. There is converted rice. How do you know what to use? Well, the long answer is that you'll have to experiment. Buy small quantities of rice at a bulk food store and try each of them to see which ones you like best. They will differ in flavor, texture and aroma. As a rule, however, if no rice variety has been specified in a recipe, use a good long-grain rice (like Thai jasmine rice); for pilafs or to serve with curries, use Indian basmati.

1 cup	**250 mL**	**white rice**
2 cups	**500 mL**	**water**

Rinse the rice in several changes of cold water (this removes excess starch and other weird things we won't mention), then drain thoroughly. Place the rice with the water into a saucepan that has a tight-fitting lid and bring to a boil over high heat. Stir once, then lower the heat to a bare simmer, put the lid on the pot and let the rice cook, undisturbed, for 15 to 20 minutes (no peeking, even).

Lift the lid and, without stirring, check to see if all the water has been absorbed and the grains are tender. If so, the rice is cooked. If not, let it cook another 5 minutes, then check again. Fluff with a fork and serve.

Makes almost 3 cups (750 mL).

Brown Rice

Brown rice is rice that's still wearing an overcoat. The outer bran layer has been left on the grain, giving it a chewier texture, a nutty flavor and more vitamins and fiber. It takes a little longer to cook, but nutritionally speaking, it's a superior food. Brown rice goes especially well with hearty stews and beans. There are many varieties of brown rice, but you're most likely to encounter long- and short-grain brown rice, and brown basmati rice. Use whichever one you like best.

| 1 cup | 250 mL | brown rice |
| 3 cups | 750 mL | water |

Using the proportions above, follow the directions for cooking white rice. The only difference will be that brown rice will take 25 to 30 minutes to cook.

Makes about 4 cups (1 L).

Wild Rice

Technically speaking, wild rice is not really rice. But let's not get into that. It looks like rice (sort of), cooks like rice (mostly), and it's delicious (definitely). It's also, however, very expensive, so we tend to use it sparingly. Which is okay, because with wild rice, a little happens to go a long way. Even just a wee bit of wild rice mixed into a plain pilaf is enough to make a person feel quite lavish. And for an all-out occasion, plain wild rice tossed with some mushrooms or sliced almonds is, well, almost too much. Dahling.

| 1 cup | 250 mL | wild rice |
| 4 cups | 1 L | water |

Using the proportions above, follow the directions for cooking white rice. It will, however, take 35 to 40 minutes (and sometimes longer, depending on the rice) to become tender. You may find that the rice will become tender before all the water has been absorbed. If this happens, just drain off the excess water before serving.

Makes 4 to 5 cups (1 L to 1.25 L).

Basic Risotto

The essential Italian comfort dish, risotto is labor-intensive, but not difficult to make. Use only arborio rice—a type of short-grain rice that becomes creamy without disintegrating. Sometimes arborio rice will be sold as "Italian style rice." Same thing. For a simply elegant meal, (dahhhling), serve this accompanied by Warm Mushroom Salad (page 62) with some Fruit Sorbet (page 204) for dessert.

5 cups	1.25 L	vegetable broth
3 tbsp.	45 mL	olive oil
1		small onion, very finely chopped
1		clove garlic, squished
1½ cups	375 mL	arborio rice
½ cup	125 mL	white wine
½ cup	125 mL	grated Parmesan cheese
		salt and pepper to taste

Heat the vegetable broth to boiling, lower the heat to the bare minimum, and keep it at a simmer.

Meanwhile, heat the olive oil in a medium-sized heavy-bottomed saucepan. Add the onion and garlic and cook, stirring over medium-low heat, until softened but not browned—6 to 8 minutes. Add the rice and cook, stirring, for 2 or 3 minutes, until it begins to look glossy, then stir in the wine and cook, continuing to stir, until it has been almost completely absorbed.

Now, here's the thing. You're going to add the simmering vegetable broth, ½ cup (125 mL) at a time, stirring constantly as each addition is absorbed by the rice. The rice will become very creamy and soft, but not mushy. If it becomes completely soft before you have used all the broth, just stop adding broth. This process should take 20 to 30 minutes.

Stir in the Parmesan cheese and season to taste with salt and pepper. Serve immediately.

Makes about 4 servings.

Risotto Add-ins

Sauté a few sliced mushrooms with the onion and garlic at the beginning of the recipe. Stir in some diced zucchini, shredded spinach or fresh peas toward the end of the cooking time. Add a diced tomato or two along with the wine.

Barley

Serve plain with a stew or stirred into a stir-fry. It has a satisfying chewy texture that can stand up to practically anything.

1 cup	**250 mL**	**barley**
3 cups	**750 mL**	**water**

In a medium saucepan, combine barley and water. Bring to a boil, then reduce heat to low, cover and cook until water is absorbed and barley is tender—about 35 to 45 minutes.

Serve immediately, seasoned with salt and pepper, or rinse under cold running water to use cold in a salad.

Makes 4 cups (1 L) cooked barley.

Quinoa

Quinoa is teeming with protein, and full of calcium. A relative newcomer to this part of the world, this grain is an ancient Inca staple. Easy to prepare, dry quinoa should be stored in the refrigerator.

1 cup	**250 mL**	**quinoa**
2 cups	**500 mL**	**water or vegetable broth**

Rinse the quinoa under cold running water, then drain. Combine with water or broth in a saucepan and bring to a boil over medium heat. Reduce heat, cover and simmer until liquid has been absorbed and grains look transparent—12 to 15 minutes. Fluff with a fork and season to taste with salt and pepper and a dab of butter.

Makes 3 cups (750 mL) cooked quinoa.

Millet

Millet has been part of the human diet for a gazillion years. It may even have been munched by dinosaurs. It cooks quickly, keeps well and is delicious.

1 cup	**250 mL**	**hulled millet**
2 ½ cups	**625 mL**	**water (or vegetable broth, for more flavor)**

Place the millet in a large, heavy skillet and stir over medium-high heat until the seeds turn golden, about 5 minutes. Remove from heat.

Combine millet with water or broth in a saucepan, and bring to a boil over high heat. Reduce heat, cover and simmer until tender and liquid has been absorbed, about 20 minutes. Remove from heat and let stand, covered, for 10 minutes before serving. Fluff with a fork and season with salt and pepper.

Makes about 3 cups (750 mL) cooked millet.

Lemon Rice

An excellent accompaniment to a curry or vegetable stew. Very lemony.

¼ cup	50 mL	butter or non-dairy margarine
½ tsp.	2 mL	salt
½ tsp.	2 mL	turmeric
		grated rind of 1 lemon
1 cup	250 mL	white long-grain rice (basmati is excellent)
		juice of 1 lemon

In a saucepan with a tightly fitting lid, melt the butter or margarine over medium heat. Add the salt, turmeric, lemon rind and rice, and sauté for 2 or 3 minutes—until the rice begins to look glassy.

Add the lemon juice combined with enough water to make 2 cups (500 mL) of liquid. Bring to a boil, then immediately lower the heat to the barest simmer and cook for about 20 minutes, until all the liquid has been absorbed, and holes appear on the surface of the rice (the surface will look slightly lunar).

Serve immediately.

Makes 3 cups (750 mL).

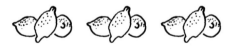

Mexican Red Rice

Make a double batch of this rice so that you'll have enough left over to stuff some Full Meal Burritos (page 166) later in the week. You'll be glad you did.

1 cup	250 mL	long-grain rice
3 tbsp.	45 mL	vegetable oil
1		small onion, chopped
1		clove garlic, squished
1 cup	250 mL	chopped, fresh or canned tomato
1 cup	250 mL	water or vegetable broth
1 cup	250 mL	cooked diced carrots or peas (or a mixture), optional
		salt and pepper to taste

Place the rice in a bowl and add hot water to cover. Let it sit while you prepare the rest of the ingredients.

Heat 1 tbsp. (15 mL) of the oil in a small saucepan over medium heat. Add the chopped onion and garlic, and let it cook for about 5 minutes, until softened. Add the chopped tomato and cook, stirring over medium-high heat for 8 to 10 minutes, until some of the liquid has evaporated. Dump the mixture into a blender or food processor along with the water or vegetable stock and blend until smooth.

Drain the rice thoroughly and rinse under cold running water until the water runs clear. Heat the remaining 2 tbsp. (30 mL) of the oil in a medium saucepan and add the drained rice. Fry, stirring from time to time, until the rice is pale golden—8 to 10 minutes. Now add the tomato mixture, let it come to a boil, then reduce the heat and cover. Let simmer for about 20 minutes over low heat, without stirring. The liquid should be absorbed and small holes will appear on the surface of the rice.

Stir in the additional vegetables, if you're using them, and let cook for an additional 5 minutes. Taste for seasoning, fluff with a fork and serve.

Makes 3 or 4 servings.

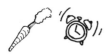

Bulgur Pilaf

Try this sturdy pilaf instead of rice, pasta or couscous. It reheats beautifully and will cheerfully wait around for the rest of dinner to be ready without going mucky.

2 tbsp.	30 mL	vegetable oil
1 cup	250 mL	bulgur wheat
1		onion, chopped
2 cups	500 mL	vegetable broth
2 tbsp.	30 mL	chopped fresh parsley
		salt and pepper to taste

Heat the oil in a medium saucepan over medium heat. Add the bulgur and the chopped onion and cook, stirring, until the onion is softened, about 5 minutes. Add the vegetable broth, parsley and salt and pepper, and bring to a boil. Lower the heat, cover and let simmer until all the water is absorbed, 20 to 25 minutes. Fluff with a fork and serve.

Makes 4 servings.

Kasha

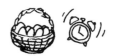

Kasha is actually buckwheat grain. You can buy it toasted or untoasted—the toasted kind (used here) is reddish brown and has a wholesome earthy flavor that can become quite addictive.

2 tbsp.	30 mL	vegetable oil
2		onions, chopped
1		egg, beaten
1 cup	250 mL	*toasted* kasha
2 cups	500 mL	vegetable broth or water
½ tsp.	2 mL	salt

Heat the vegetable oil in a medium saucepan, add the chopped onions and sauté over medium heat until golden. Remove the onions from the pan and set aside.

In a small bowl, stir together the beaten egg and the kasha. Scoop the mixture into the same saucepan in which you cooked the onions—don't add any additional oil. Cook, stirring to break up clumps, until the egg has dried and the grains are separate and beginning to brown.

Pour in the vegetable broth or water and bring the mixture to a boil. Add the sautéed onions, cover and cook over low heat for 20 to 25 minutes, until the kasha is tender and the liquid has been absorbed.

Serve just the way it is, as a side dish. You can't beat it for soaking up sauce.

Makes about 4 servings.

Extra Added Attraction

Toss the cooked kasha with an equal volume of cooked egg noodles or bow-tie pasta for a traditional touch. Really. A few sautéed mushrooms wouldn't hurt either.

Multigrain Pilaf

Serve this delicious pilaf as a side dish, or bake it in a halved acorn or other small winter squash. Add other cooked grains—like wheat berries or millet—if you like, or toss in a can of drained beans to turn it into a main dish.

2 cups	500 mL	cooked brown rice (page 169)
1 cup	250 mL	cooked wild rice (page 169)
1 cup	250 mL	cooked barley (page 171)
1 cup	250 mL	cooked corn niblets—from fresh, frozen or canned
½ cup	125 mL	raisins or dried cranberries
2 tbsp.	30 mL	butter or non-dairy margarine
½ cup	125 mL	chopped pecans
		salt and pepper to taste

In a large bowl, toss together the brown rice, wild rice, barley, corn niblets and raisins or cranberries.

Melt the non-dairy margarine in a small skillet, add the chopped pecans, and cook over medium-low heat, stirring, until lightly toasted—about 5 minutes. Add to the rice mixture, and toss very well. Season to taste with salt and pepper and dump into a greased casserole dish. Cover and bake at 350° F (180° C) for 20 to 25 minutes, until heated through.

Makes 4 to 6 servings.

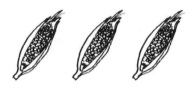

Baked Stuffed Squash

Buy any small winter squash—like acorn or pepper squash, delicata squash or small buttercup squash. One medium squash will make 1 or 2 servings.

Remove the stem, cut each squash in half lengthwise and scoop out the seeds. Place the squash halves into a baking dish, cut side down, and pour a little water into the bottom to about ¼-inch (.5 cm) deep. Bake at 425° F (220° C) for 20 minutes. Turn the squash halves over in the baking dish, brush the cut surfaces liberally with melted butter or olive oil, then:

- Fill the cavity of the squash halves with Multigrain Pilaf (opposite); or
- Stuff with your favorite chili and sprinkle with shredded cheese; or
- Scoop in some leftover macaroni and cheese; or
- Fill with any cooked vegetable mixture; or
- Drizzle with maple syrup.

Then return to the oven and bake for another 15 to 20 minutes, until the squash is completely tender and the filling (if any) is heated through.

Vegetables on the Side

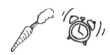

Ratatouille

Ratatouille is a very adaptable dish. You can, of course, serve it as a side dish, either hot or at room temperature. Or you can serve it as a main course with pasta or rice, or rolled into crepes.

2 tbsp.	30 mL	olive or vegetable oil
1		medium onion, chopped
4		cloves garlic, squished
1		medium eggplant, peeled and cut into ½-inch (1 cm) cubes
2		medium zucchini, cut into ½-inch (1 cm) cubes
2		medium green or red peppers, diced
¼ cup	50 mL	chopped fresh basil (or 1 tbsp./15 mL dried)
2 cups	500 mL	diced canned tomatoes (or about 4 medium fresh tomatoes, chopped)
½ tsp.	2 mL	salt
¼ tsp.	1 mL	pepper

Heat the olive oil in a very large skillet or Dutch oven over medium heat and cook the onion and garlic until soft—about 5 minutes. Add the eggplant, zucchini, peppers and basil. Mix well, and cook, stirring, for 10 minutes, until vegetables are almost tender. Add the tomatoes, salt and pepper, and cook for about 15 minutes more, stirring occasionally, until the vegetables are tender and the flavors are blended.

Serve hot or at room temperature.

Makes about 8 servings as a side dish or 4 as a main course.

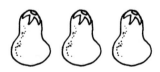

Red Cabbage with Apples

Try this for a perfect fall dinner: Baked Stuffed Squash (page 177), Multigrain Pilaf (page 176) and Red Cabbage with Apples.

3 tbsp.	45 mL	vegetable oil
2		medium onions, chopped
1		small head red cabbage, cut into shreds
2		apples, chopped (you don't have to peel them)
½ cup	125 mL	red wine (any kind—even leftover yucky stuff is okay)
¼ cup	50 mL	apple cider vinegar (or any vinegar)
1 tbsp.	15 mL	sugar
2 tsp.	10 mL	salt
½ cup	125 mL	red currant jelly

In a very large pot (that has a lid) heat the oil over medium heat. Add the onions and cook, stirring for 5 minutes, until softened. Add the cabbage and cook, over medium-low heat, for 10 to 15 minutes— until the cabbage is softened. Now add the apples, wine, vinegar, sugar and salt, lower the heat to a simmer and cook, covered for 1½ to 2 hours, stirring occasionally. (Go do something useful, like read a book or eat cookies.)

Stir in the red currant jelly, cover and simmer for another 15 to 20 minutes.

Makes 8-ish very colorful servings.

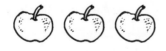

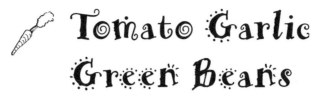

Tomato Garlic Green Beans

Here's an exception to the never-overcook-vegetables rule. The beans in this dish should be cooked until tender and squishy and totally infused with the flavor of the sauce. It's a great use for those green beans that have seen better days (you know—the ones at the back of your refrigerator). Try this with Old-Fashioned Potato Soup (page 45) and Sweet and Sour Roasted Beet Salad (page 59), and a lot of good bread.

2 tbsp.	30 mL	olive oil
1		large onion, chopped
2		cloves garlic, squished
1 lb.	500 g	diced, peeled tomatoes
1 lb.	500 g	fresh green beans, cut into 1-inch (2 cm) pieces
1 tsp.	5 mL	crumbled oregano
1 tsp.	5 mL	salt
¼ tsp.	1 mL	pepper

Heat the oil in a large skillet over medium heat. Add the onion and garlic, and sauté until they are soft and lightly golden—about 10 minutes. Add the tomatoes and bring to a simmer, stirring occasionally. Now, stir in the green beans and oregano, cover and simmer for about 30 minutes, stirring a few times, until the beans are quite soft. Add salt and pepper, cook for another minute or two, and serve.

Makes 4 to 6 servings, as a side dish.

Oven-Roasted Vegetables

Vary this recipe to use whatever vegetables you happen to have—just make sure the veggies are cut into big chunky pieces so that they don't cook too quickly. You can serve these plain as a side dish, tossed with pasta or rice, or cooled to room temperature and drizzled with balsamic vinegar as a salad.

2		sweet potatoes, peeled
1		large Spanish onion (or 2 smaller ones)
1		large sweet red pepper
½ lb.	250 g	fresh mushrooms
1		medium zucchini
¼ cup	50 mL	olive oil
1 tbsp.	15 mL	fresh rosemary (or 1 tsp./5 mL dried)
½ tsp.	2 mL	salt

Trim all the vegetables, removing stems or cores or whatever they happen to have, and cut into 1-inch (2.5 cm) chunks. If the mushrooms are very large, cut them in half, otherwise leave them whole. Place everything in a bowl and toss with the olive oil, rosemary and salt.

Spread the vegetables out in a large baking pan—like a big lasagne pan—so that they are in a single layer. They need room to brown properly. Bake at 425° F (220° C) for 40 to 45 minutes, tossing around occasionally, until all the vegetables are tender and very well browned.

Makes about 4 servings.

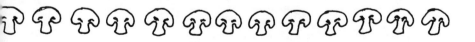

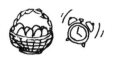

Potato Kugel

Although this is often served as a side dish in a non-vegetarian meal, it's really substantial enough to be a main course.

6		large potatoes, peeled
1		large onion
4		eggs
1 tsp.	5 mL	salt
¼ tsp.	1 mL	pepper (or to taste)
¼ cup	50 mL	chopped fresh parsley (if you have it)
6 tbsp.	90 mL	flour
6 tbsp.	90 mL	vegetable oil

Grate the potatoes into a large mixing bowl using either the large holes of a hand grater or the shredding blade of a food processor. Dump the grated potatoes into a colander and run cold water over them—this keeps them from going black. Really. Drain well, squeezing out as much water as possible, and return them to the mixing bowl.

Grate or chop the onion very finely and add to the shredded potatoes. Beat the eggs with the salt and pepper, and add to the potato mixture along with the chopped parsley. Sprinkle in the flour and mix the whole thing up thoroughly.

Now pour the oil into a 9 x 13-inch (22 x 33 cm) rectangular baking dish and put it into the oven. Turn the oven on to 375° F (190° C) and let the oil heat for about 5 minutes. Remove the baking dish from the oven and pour most of the hot oil into the potato mixture, leaving just a little in the bottom of the baking dish. Stir well and plop the whole business into the baking dish. Bake for 1 hour until the top is nicely browned and crisp.

Makes about 12 servings.

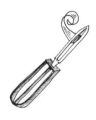

Spicy Corn

*There's only so much plain corn on the cob a person can eat before
you begin to feel the urge to mess with it. A little garlic, a little
cayenne and a splodge of cream should do the trick.*

4		cobs fresh corn
3 tbsp.	45 mL	butter
2		cloves garlic, squished
¼ tsp.	1 mL	cayenne (or more, if you dare)
½ tsp.	2 mL	salt
½ cup	125 mL	milk (or, to be truly decadent, cream)

With a sharp knife, cut the corn kernels off the cobs, scraping the
cobs to remove as much of the pulp as possible.

Melt the butter in a medium skillet, add the corn kernels, garlic,
cayenne and salt, and cook for 5 or 6 minutes, until the corn is tender but still crisp. Add the milk or cream and let simmer for another
5 or 6 minutes, until the sauce is creamy and the corn is cooked.

Makes 2 or 3 servings.

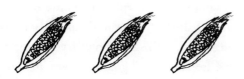

Fried Bananas or Plantains

And now for something completely different. For a tropical dinner, serve this with Cuban-Style Black Beans (page 139), Orange and Red Onion Salad (page 64), white rice and some hot Latin music.

4		large green bananas or ripe plantains (if you can get them)
½ cup	125 mL	flour
½ tsp.	2 mL	salt
¼ tsp.	1 mL	pepper
		vegetable oil for frying

Peel the bananas or plantains and cut into ¼-inch (.5 cm) diagonal slices.

In a bowl or on a piece of waxed paper, combine the flour, salt and pepper. Toss each piece of banana or plantain in the flour mixture to coat lightly.

Meanwhile, pour enough vegetable oil into a large frying pan just to cover the bottom of the pan evenly. Place on the stove over medium heat. When a drop of water in the pan begins to sizzle, arrange the bananas or plantains in a single layer in the hot skillet. Let cook for 2 to 4 minutes, until golden brown, then turn each piece over and allow the other side to cook until golden. Using a spatula or pancake turner, carefully remove from the pan onto a warm plate. You may have to do this in batches unless you have a huge frying pan. Add a little more oil to the pan, if necessary, between batches.

Serve hot, with a little hot pepper sauce on the side.

Makes 4 servings.

Lentil Dal

Dal is the general name for an Indian dish made from lentils or some other type of legume. It's usually fairly soupy and can be served alone with rice, or as part of an Indian dinner. You can even roll it into a warm flour tortilla for a quick meal on the run. Try it with Cauliflower Curry (page 130), Indian Vegetable Pilau (page 151) and a Raita (page 131).

1 cup	250 mL	dry lentils
4 cups	1 L	water
1 tsp.	5 mL	salt
2 tbsp.	30 mL	finely grated fresh ginger root
½ tsp.	2 mL	turmeric
¼ tsp.	1 mL	ground cardamom
¼ tsp.	1 mL	cayenne
2 tbsp.	30 mL	vegetable oil (or butter)
½ tsp.	2 mL	hot pepper flakes
½ tsp.	2 mL	ground cumin
2 tbsp.	30 mL	chopped cilantro
2 tbsp.	30 mL	lemon juice

Rinse the lentils, then place them in a medium saucepan with the water and salt. Bring to a boil over medium heat, then lower the heat, cover, and let the lentils simmer for 1 hour, stirring occasionally. Add the ginger, turmeric, cardamom and cayenne, and continue to simmer until the lentils are completely soft, adding a bit more water if necessary (the mixture should be like a thick soup).

Meanwhile, add the vegetable oil or melt the butter in a small skillet over medium heat. Add the hot pepper flakes and the cumin and cook, stirring, for 2 or 3 minutes. Add this mixture to the lentils, along with the chopped cilantro and the lemon juice. Serve hot.

Makes 4 to 6 servings.

8. Baked Stuff

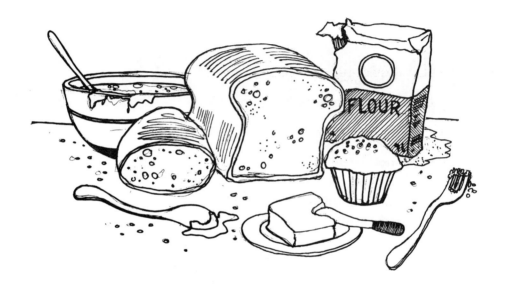

Ultra-Quick All-Purpose Yeast Dough

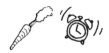

Who has time to hang around waiting for dough to rise? Not you. This easy recipe will let you whip up a pizza crust, a slab of focaccia or a fabulous loaf of bread, and still have a life. The secret is something called "quick-rise instant yeast" (available everywhere, alongside regular yeast granules) which does the job in about half the time of the ordinary stuff.

3½ cups	875 mL	all-purpose flour
1 tbsp.	15 mL	"quick-rise" dry yeast granules (1 envelope)
1 tsp.	5 mL	salt
1 cup	250 mL	hot tap water
2 tbsp.	30 mL	olive or vegetable oil

In a large bowl, stir together 2 cups (500 mL) of the flour, the yeast granules and the salt. Add the hot water and oil, and stir until the mixture is smooth (it will be sticky and gooey—don't worry). Now add the rest of the flour, ½ cup (125 mL) at a time, stirring it with a wooden spoon until it starts to become hard to stir.

At this point, dump about ½ cup (125 mL) of the flour onto your counter or table, spread it around a bit, then turn the sticky lump of dough out onto this floured surface. Begin kneading the dough by hand, adding only as much extra flour as is necessary to keep it from sticking to your hands (or the table). Continue to knead for at least 8 to 10 minutes, until the dough is no longer sticky and the surface is smooth and pliable (it will feel like your earlobe—really).

Place the dough into a large, oiled bowl. Turn it over to make sure all the sides of the dough are oiled, then cover with plastic wrap and place in a warmish place to rise. It could take anywhere from 20 to 40 minutes for the dough to rise to double in size, depending on complex cosmic factors. Be patient.

When the dough has doubled, punch it down to deflate it, then knead it a few times. Let rest for 5 minutes, and use to make pizza (page 152) or focaccia (page 190).

Makes enough dough for two 12-inch (30 cm) pizzas, or 2 pans of focaccia.

Oatmeal Raisin Bread

The essential breakfast bread.

5–6 cups	1.25–1.5 L	all-purpose white flour
2½ cups	625 mL	quick-cooking (not instant) rolled oats
¼ cup	50 mL	brown sugar
4½ tsp.	22 mL	quick-rise instant yeast (2 envelopes)
2 tsp.	10 mL	salt
1½ cups	375 mL	water
1¼ cups	300 mL	soy milk or milk
¼ cup	50 mL	vegetable oil
½ cup	125 mL	raisins, soaked in boiling water and drained

In a very large bowl, stir together 3 cups (750 mL) of the flour, the oats, brown sugar, yeast and salt. In a small saucepan, combine the water, soy milk, raisins and oil, and heat until just hot to the touch. Add the liquids to the flour mixture and stir until everything is well combined. Now, add the remaining flour, ½ cup (125 mL) at a time, until the dough becomes too stiff to stir in the bowl. It will still be pretty sticky at this point.

Now sprinkle a generous amount of flour on your table or counter and turn the dough out onto this surface. Sprinkle the dough with plenty of flour too, and begin to knead. Keep kneading the dough, sprinkling it with flour, for about 10 minutes—until it no longer sticks to your hands or the counter and is fairly smooth. (The oats will make it a little bumpy). Place the dough in an oiled bowl, turning it over so that it's oiled all over, and put into a warm place to rise until doubled in size—about 30 minutes.

Remove the dough from the bowl and punch your fist into it to deflate. Knead the dough a couple of times and—*ta da!*—it's time to make your loaves. Cut the dough in half and form into two loaves. Place each one in a well-greased loaf pan. Let the breads rise again until almost doubled—20 to 30 minutes.

Preheat the oven to 375° F (190° C). Brush the tops of the loaves with a little warm water, sprinkle with a few flakes of rolled oats (or whatever) and bake for 35 to 45 minutes, or until deep golden brown. Remove from pans, and let cool for at least a few minutes before devouring.

Makes 2 gorgeous loaves which, incidentally, happen to make great toast. If there's any left.

Fabulous Focaccia

You can load your focaccia down with toppings, or just leave it simple. Whatever you do, it'll be great. Serve this as an accompaniment to a bowl of Phenomenal Minestrone Soup (page 48) or Creamy Carrot Soup (page 44).

1 recipe		ultra-quick all-purpose yeast dough
¼ cup	50 mL	olive or vegetable oil
2		onions, sliced
4		cloves garlic, squished
¼ cup	50 mL	grated Parmesan cheese (optional)
1 tsp.	5 mL	crumbled dried rosemary or oregano
½ tsp.	2 mL	salt
¼ tsp.	1 mL	pepper

Divide the dough into 2 pieces. Working with one piece at a time, flatten it out into an 8-inch (20 cm) circle, about ½-inch (1 cm) thick. Place on a greased baking sheet. Repeat with the remaining dough.

Heat the oil in a large skillet over medium heat. Add the onions and garlic, and cook, stirring occasionally, until softened—5 to 7 minutes. Remove from heat and let cool for a few minutes. Divide the onion mixture between the two rounds of dough, spreading it out almost to the edges. Sprinkle with the Parmesan, rosemary or oregano, salt and pepper.

Let the breads rise in a warm place for 20 to 30 minutes, until a little puffy.

Bake at 375° F (190° C) for 20 to 25 minutes, until the bottom of the focaccia is lightly browned, and the top crust is golden. Eat while still warm, if possible.

Makes two 10-inch (30 cm) breads.

A Simple Focaccia

Make little indentations all over the surface of the risen dough with your fingertips, brush liberally with olive oil, and sprinkle with coarse salt, fresh ground pepper and crumbled rosemary. Bake as for Fabulous Focaccia.

Jalapeño Cornbread

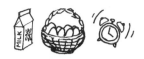

*If there's a better accompaniment to a bowl of Veggie-Packed Chili
(page 126), I don't know what it could possibly be.*

1½ cups	375 mL	white flour
1 cup	250 mL	yellow cornmeal
2 tbsp.	30 mL	sugar
2 tbsp.	30 mL	baking powder
1 tsp.	5 mL	salt
¼ cup	50 mL	vegetable oil
1		egg
1⅓ cups	325 mL	milk or soy milk
¼ cup	50 mL	chopped fresh (or canned) jalapeño peppers
½ tsp.	2 mL	hot pepper flakes (optional—use if you want some real heat)

Measure the flour, cornmeal, sugar, baking powder and salt into a
large bowl and stir to mix. In a smaller bowl, beat together the oil,
egg and milk. Now pour the milk mixture into the flour mixture, and
stir together with a wooden spoon until pretty well combined. A few
lumps are okay—resist the temptation to overbeat. Fold in the
chopped jalapeño peppers and the hot pepper flakes (if you're using
them).

Pour batter into a well-greased 8-inch (20 cm) square baking pan,
smooshing the top so that it's even. Bake at 350° F (180° C) for 20 to
25 minutes, or until a toothpick poked into the middle comes out
clean. Let cool for just a couple of minutes before cutting into
squares, then serve while still warm.

Makes about 9 big hunks of cornbread, or lots more small ones.

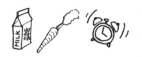

Homemade Biscuit Mix

This biscuit mix can be used in any recipe that calls for commercial biscuit mix to make biscuits, quick breads or pancakes. It can be kept almost forever at room temperature—and even longer in the refrigerator.

8½ cups	2 L	flour (all-purpose white or half white and half whole wheat)
3 tbsp.	45 mL	baking powder
2 tsp.	10 mL	salt
2 tsp.	10 mL	cream of tartar
1 tsp.	5 mL	baking soda
1½ cups	375 mL	skim milk powder or soy milk powder
1 lb.	500 g	solid vegetable shortening (like Crisco)

In a huge bowl, stir together all the dry ingredients until you're sure they're well mixed. Using a pastry blender, cut the shortening into the flour mixture until it resembles coarse cornmeal. This can also be done in batches in a food processor—just make sure you divide the ingredients equally, and don't overprocess the mixture. It should remain mealy.

Store the mixture at room temperature or in the refrigerator in a tightly covered container, and use in any recipe that calls for commercial biscuit mix.

Makes about 10 cups (2.5 L) biscuit mix.

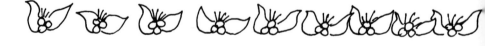

Biscuits From Scratch (or not)

From scratch:

2 cups	500 mL	all-purpose flour (or half all-purpose and half whole wheat)
4 tsp.	20 mL	baking powder
½ tsp.	2 mL	salt
1 tbsp.	15 mL	sugar (optional—use for a sweet biscuit)
½ cup	125 mL	butter, margarine or solid vegetable shortening
¾ cup	175 mL	milk or soy milk

From mix:

2 cups	500 mL	biscuit mix—homemade (opposite), or commercial
½ cup	125 mL	milk, water or soy milk

If you are making your biscuits from scratch, stir together the flour, baking powder, salt and sugar, if using, in a mixing bowl. With a pastry blender or two knives, cut in the butter (or shortening) until the mixture is crumbly and resembles coarse cornmeal. Add the milk, stirring until the mixture is combined and can be gathered together into a ball of dough.

If you are using biscuit mix, stir together the mix with whatever liquid you're using, just until it forms a soft dough.

Gently roll or pat the dough out to about ½-inch (1 cm) thickness. Cut biscuits out with a 2-inch (5 cm) round cookie cutter (or a drinking glass dipped in flour). Place biscuits on an ungreased cookie sheet and bake at 425° F (220° C) for 10 to 12 minutes, until lightly browned.

If you're not in the mood to mess around, or if, for some reason, your dough is too soft to roll out, simply scoop spoonfuls of the dough out onto an ungreased cookie sheet and bake as above.

Makes 10 to 12 biscuits.

Parmesan Onion Bread

A good snack bread for eating by itself, or to serve with a bowl of soup. Great with a bowl of Pasta Fagioli (page 52).

2 cups	500 mL	flour
1 tbsp.	15 mL	baking powder
½ tsp.	2 mL	salt
¼ cup	50 mL	butter or shortening
¾ cup	175 mL	milk
1		small onion, chopped
½ cup	125 mL	grated Parmesan cheese
½ cup	125 mL	mayonnaise
1 tbsp.	30 mL	finely chopped jalapeño pepper (optional, but good)

In a bowl, stir together the flour, baking powder and salt. With a pastry blender (or using two knives) cut the butter or shortening into the flour mixture until it resembles coarse crumbs. Add the milk and stir to make a soft dough. By hand, squash the dough evenly into a greased 8- or 9-inch (20 or 22 cm) square baking pan, covering the entire bottom.

In another bowl, stir together the onion, Parmesan cheese, mayonnaise and jalapeño pepper (if you're using them). Spread this stuff evenly over the dough in the pan.

Bake at 400° F (200° C) for 15 to 20 minutes, until very lightly browned on the edges.

Cut into squares and serve while still warm.

Makes 6 to 8 servings.

Ridiculously Easy Cheese Quickbread

This quickbread doesn't need kneading or rising. Whatever you don't eat right away can be sliced to make a super sandwich.

2 cups	500 mL	flour
4 tsp.	20 mL	baking powder
1 tbsp.	15 mL	sugar
½ tsp.	2 mL	dry mustard powder
½ tsp.	2 mL	salt
1¼ cups	300 mL	shredded cheese (Cheddar, Monterey Jack, Swiss)
1		egg
1 cup	250 mL	milk
2 tbsp.	15 mL	vegetable oil

In a large bowl, stir together the flour, baking powder, sugar, mustard powder, salt and cheese until thoroughly combined.

In a smaller bowl, beat the egg with the milk and the vegetable oil. All at once, pour the egg mixture into the flour mixture and stir just until all the ingredients are moistened. The batter will be lumpy—but that's okay.

Preheat the oven to 375°F (190°C). Spoon batter into a greased loaf pan and bake for 45 to 50 minutes—or until the top is beginning to brown lightly. Allow bread to cool for about 10 minutes before attempting to remove from the pan.

Makes one ridiculously easy loaf.

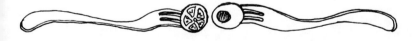

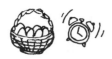

Banana Oat Muffins

These muffins are a dignified finale for those poor black bananas that have been festering on your counter all week.

¾ cup	175 mL	all-purpose flour
½ cup	125 mL	quick-cooking rolled oats (not instant)
½ cup	125 mL	sugar
1 tsp.	5 mL	baking soda
½ tsp.	2 mL	baking powder
½ cup	125 mL	vegetable oil
2		medium-sized ripe bananas
2		eggs

In a large bowl, stir together the flour, oats, sugar, baking soda and baking powder.

In the container of a blender or food processor, blend together the oil, bananas and eggs until really smooth. Pour the banana mixture into the flour mixture and stir just until combined.

Spoon batter into a well-greased muffin pan, filling the cups almost to the top. Bake at 375° F (190° C) for 25 to 30 minutes.

Makes about 9 muffins.

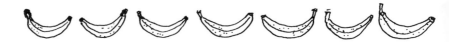

Carrot Apple Muffins

Not too sweet, not too cakey—these muffins are a very cheery way to start your morning.

2		eggs
½ cup	125 mL	sugar
1 tsp.	5 mL	vanilla extract
½ cup	125 mL	plain yogurt
¼ cup	50 mL	vegetable oil
1 cup	250 mL	all-purpose flour (or half all-purpose and half whole wheat)
1 tsp.	5 mL	baking soda
½ tsp.	2 mL	cinnamon
¾ cup	175 mL	shredded scrubbed carrot (about 1 medium carrot)
¾ cup	175 mL	shredded peeled and cored apple (about 1 medium apple)
½ cup	125 mL	chopped walnuts

In a medium bowl, beat together the eggs, sugar and vanilla until very well mixed. Add the yogurt and vegetable oil, and beat well.

In a small bowl, stir together the flour, baking soda and cinnamon. Add to the egg mixture, stir until smooth, then add the shredded carrot and apple, and the chopped nuts. Stir just until combined.

Spoon batter into a well-greased muffin pan, filling the cups almost all the way to the top. Bake at 375° F (190° C) for 20 to 25 minutes, until a toothpick poked into the middle of a muffin comes out clean.

Makes about 9 muffins.

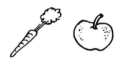

9. Just Desserts

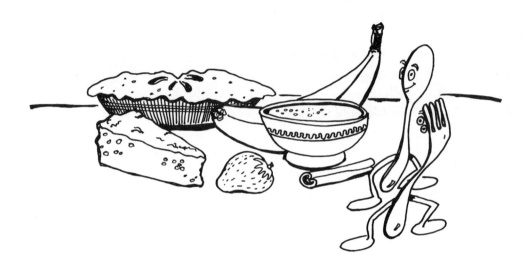

Amazing Eggless Dairy-Free Chocolate Cake

Just because you don't use eggs or dairy doesn't mean you shouldn't have your chocolate cake (and eat it too). This one is so perfectly normal, so absolutely delicious, no one will believe how easy it is to make.

1½ cups	375 mL	flour
1 cup	250 mL	sugar
¼ cup	50 mL	unsweetened cocoa powder
1 tsp.	5 mL	baking soda
1 tsp.	5 mL	vinegar
1 tsp.	5 mL	vanilla extract
⅓ cup	75 mL	vegetable oil
1 cup	250 mL	water

In a medium bowl, stir together the flour, sugar, cocoa powder and baking soda until well mixed. All at once add the vinegar, vanilla, oil and water. Stir well, then dump the batter into a well-greased 8-inch (20 cm) square baking pan. Bake at 350° F (180° C) for 30 to 35 minutes, until a toothpick poked into the center of the cake comes out clean.

Let cool completely before frosting (if desired).

Now what could possibly be easier?

Make one 8-inch (20 cm) cake.

Amazing Eggless Dairy-Free Orange Cake

Double the recipe if you want to make a two-layer cake. Bake it in two well-greased 9-inch (22 cm) round cake pans for the same amount of time.

1½ cups	375 mL	flour
¾ cup	175 mL	sugar
1 tsp.	5 mL	baking soda
½ tsp.	2 mL	baking powder
1 cup	250 mL	orange juice
⅓ cup	75 mL	vegetable oil
1 tsp.	5 mL	grated orange rind

In a medium bowl, stir together the flour, sugar, baking soda and baking powder until well mixed. All at once, add the orange juice, vegetable oil and orange rind. Stir just enough to combine the ingredients, then immediately dump into a well-greased 8-inch (20 cm) square baking dish. Resist the urge to overstir the batter—you'll only deflate it. Bake at 350° F (180° C) for 35 to 40 minutes, or until a toothpick poked into the middle of the cake comes out clean, and the cake is lightly browned on top.

Cool completely before slathering it with icing (if that's what you plan to do) or burying it under fresh fruit.

Makes one 8-inch (20 cm) cake.

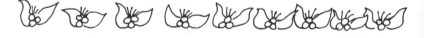

Two Fabulous Frostings

Look for the word "pareve" on the package when you're shopping for margarine. That tells you the margarine contains no milk ingredients whatsoever and can be eaten by vegetarians who do not use dairy products.

Non-Dairy Chocolate Frosting

1 cup	250 mL	non-dairy "pareve" margarine
½ cup	125 mL	unsweetened cocoa powder
½ tsp.	2 mL	vanilla extract
2 cups	500 mL	icing sugar (powdered confectioner's sugar)

In a food processor, or in a large bowl with an electric mixer, beat the margarine until smooth and creamy. Add the cocoa, vanilla and icing sugar, and beat until very smooth and fluffy.

Makes enough icing for a two-layer cake.

Non-Dairy Vanilla Frosting

1 cup	250 mL	non-dairy "pareve" margarine
1 tsp.	5 mL	vanilla extract
3 cups	750 mL	icing sugar (powdered confectioner's sugar)

In a food processor, or in a large bowl with an electric mixer, beat the margarine until very smooth and creamy. Add the vanilla and the icing sugar. Continue beating until smooth and fluffy. If the icing is too thick, you can add up to 2 tbsp. (30 mL) orange juice or soy milk to thin it, a few drops at a time.

Makes enough icing for a two-layer cake.

Fruit Crisp

Use whatever fruit is in season to make a delicious fruit crisp. You can even use frozen fruit (if that's all you have) or make it with a mixture of wrinkly odds and ends.

6 cups	1.5 L	prepared fruit (see below)
½ cup	125 mL	sugar
3 tbsp.	45 mL	cornstarch
1 cup	250 mL	flour
½ cup	125 mL	non-dairy margarine (or butter)
½ cup	125 mL	brown sugar
½ tsp.	2 mL	cinnamon (optional, depending on the fruit)

In a large bowl, toss the fruit—whatever you're using—with the sugar and cornstarch. Feel free to adjust the amount of sugar to suit your taste and the type of fruit—it won't affect the results. Dump into a greased 8- or 9-inch (20 or 22 cm) square baking dish.

In a food processor, or in a bowl with a fork or pastry blender, combine the flour, butter or margarine, brown sugar and cinnamon. Mix and mash until the mixture becomes moist and crumbly. Sprinkle evenly over the top of the fruit in the baking dish. Bake at 375° F (190° F) for 35 to 45 minutes, until the fruit is bubbly and the topping is browned.

Serve warm with regular or tofu ice cream, frozen yogurt or whipped cream.

Makes 6 to 8 servings.

Fruit Ideas

- *Peeled, cored and sliced apples or pears*
- *Peeled, pitted and sliced peaches*
- *Diced rhubarb*
- *Blueberries, strawberries or raspberries*
- *Pitted and quartered plums*
- *Tutti fruitti—a little of this and a little of that!*

Seemingly Normal Chocolate Pudding

The original comfort dessert, ever-so-slightly adjusted to eliminate dairy products. Still very comforting.

1¼ cups	300 mL	sugar
½ cup	125 mL	unsweetened cocoa powder
3 tbsp.	45 mL	cornstarch
2½ cups	625 mL	soy milk
¼ cup	50 mL	non-dairy margarine or butter
2 tsp.	10 mL	vanilla extract

In a medium saucepan, stir together the sugar, cocoa powder and the cornstarch. Add just enough soy milk to the mixture to make a thick paste, then stir in the rest of the soy milk. Cook over medium-low heat, stirring almost constantly, until the mixture thickens and gets bubbly. Reduce the heat to low and continue to cook for another minute or two, then remove from heat and stir in the margarine and vanilla.

Pour into serving dishes, covering the surface with plastic wrap to prevent a skin from forming on top, and refrigerate. Chill thoroughly before serving.

Makes 6 to 8 seemingly normal servings.

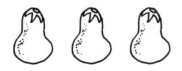

Fabulous Fresh Fruit Sorbet

This sorbet can be made with almost any kind of fruit, or with lemon or orange juice, or even with canned fruit—like pineapple. The flavor will knock your socks off. Try making this with fresh strawberries, raspberries, mangoes, peaches or melons for a killer summer dessert.

1 cup	250 mL	water
½ cup	125 mL	sugar
2 cups	500 mL	puréed fresh fruit
2 tbsp.	30 mL	lemon juice

In a small saucepan, bring the water and sugar to a boil over medium-high heat, stirring only until the sugar is dissolved. Let this mixture cook for exactly 5 minutes (timing from the minute it came to a boil), then remove from heat and let cool to room temperature.

Stir together the puréed fruit, the sugar mixture and the lemon juice. Pour this mixture into an aluminum (or stainless steel) 8-inch (20 cm) square baking dish. Place in the freezer and let it freeze until solid—3 to 4 hours. Remove the frozen mixture from the pan, break it into chunks, and purée in a food processor until smooth and creamy. Dump into a container and return to the freezer for about 30 minutes, or until you're ready to serve it.

Serve garnished with some fresh berries or a few mint leaves. Amazing.

Makes 3 or 4 servings.

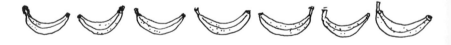

Fruit Compote

You had a good reason for buying that basket of peaches/apples/pears/whatever. Only now you can't remember what it was. And—yikes—they're all-too-quickly decomposing on your counter. Quick! Make some compote!

6 cups	1.5 L	prepared fruit
½ cup	125 mL	sugar (or less, to taste)
1		cinnamon stick

Rummage through your fruit and cut out any squishy or rotten parts. Peel everything, then cut into slices or chunks—whatever works. You can use apples, peaches, plums, pears, cherries, nectarines—practically anything. Any mixture of fruit will do.

Dump fruit into a saucepan with the sugar and a cinnamon stick. Let sit at room temperature for about an hour to draw out the juices, then bring to a boil over medium-low heat. Cook, stirring gently— don't mash the fruit—for about 10 minutes, until everything is tender. Cool to room temperature, then chill.

Serve compote in a pretty glass dish, either plain or with a dollop of yogurt or whipped cream. Or spoon it over a slab of cake.

Makes about 6 servings.

More Quickie Vegan Dessert Ideas

- Soy milk can be used in place of regular milk in *most* dessert recipes, like pudding or cakes.
- Fruit pies are usually made with vegetable shortening so you should be okay. Skip the ice cream, or use tofu ice cream instead.
- Bake shortbread cookies with non-dairy "pareve" margarine instead of butter. If you are desperate for decadence, you can use non-dairy whipped topping. Make sure you look for the word "pareve" on the label, or it *may* contain some dairy ingredients.
- Dip fresh fruit in warm chocolate sauce for a delicious fruit fondue.
- Look for fruit sorbets or water ices made without milk.
- Buy kosher gelatin, which is vegetable-based, instead of regular gelatin.

Peach and Banana Flambé

There's nothing like a flaming dessert to wake up your dinner guests. Be sure to prepare this in front of everyone for full dramatic effect.

3		medium bananas
2		large peaches
1 tbsp.	15 mL	lemon juice
¼ cup	50 mL	non-dairy "pareve" margarine or butter
⅔ cup	150 mL	brown sugar
¼ cup	50 mL	light rum or banana (or whatever) liqueur

Peel the bananas and cut, crosswise, into diagonal slices, about ½-inch (1 cm) thick. Peel the peaches, remove the pits and slice thickly. Place the bananas and peaches in a bowl and toss with the lemon juice.

In a large skillet, melt the butter or margarine over medium-high heat. Stir in the brown sugar. Add the bananas and peaches to the pan and cook, stirring gently so as not to mash the fruit, for 3 or 4 minutes, until glazed and bubbly. Pour in the rum, stir and heat until it almost simmers. Remove from heat and immediately ignite it with a match. It should flame very impressively for a couple of minutes and then die out. Make sure everyone sees this, then serve over slices of cake or with regular or tofu ice cream. Or both.

Very fancy.

Makes 4 servings.

Truly Astonishing Tofu Chocolate Mousse

No really—this is amazing. It has to be tried to be believed.

1 package		(19 oz./539 g) silken tofu
2 cups	500 mL	chocolate chips

Dump the tofu into the container of a food processor or blender and blend until smooth, scraping down the sides once or twice.

Melt the chocolate chips in a small saucepan set into another saucepan filled with boiling water (or in a double boiler), stirring until smooth. Pour the melted chocolate into the blender or processor and blend until the mixture is very smooth and creamy. Spoon into individual dessert dishes and chill. Serve plain or with a dollop of whipped cream.

Makes about 6 very surprising servings.

Extra Added Attraction!

Use this mousse to fill a baked pie shell (or a graham cracker crust) for an amazing, decadent chocolate mousse pie. Top it, if you want, with non-dairy whipped topping or real whipped cream, and sprinkle with shaved chocolate.

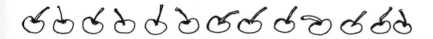

index

A

African Peanut Soup, 54
alfalfa sprouts, 118
All-Purpose Tomato Pasta
  Sauce, 95-96
Amazing Eggless Dairy-Free
  Chocolate Cake, 199
Amazing Eggless Dairy-Free
  Orange Cake, 200
appetizers
  artichokes, 32
  Baba Ghanouj, 29
  Chunky Avocado Salsa,
    24
  Fresh Tomato Salsa, 26
  Homemade Refried
    Beans, 36
  Hummus, 23
  Mexican Meltdown, 31
  Muncho Grande Platter,
    37
  polenta, 141
  Quesadillas, 35
  Roasted Garlic, 30
  Salsa Cheese Bites, 33
  Spanakopita triangles,
    149
  Spicy Black Bean Dip, 27
  Tzatziki, 28
  Veggie Paté, 32
  Zucchini Appetizers, 34
artichokes, 32
asparagus
  Spicy Oriental Asparagus
    Salad, 76
Authentic Greek Salad, 66
avocados, 24
  Chunky Avocado Salsa,
    24
  plant project, 25

B

Baba Ghanouj, 29
Baked Barbecue Tofu Steaks,
  156
Baked Broccoli Egg Squares,
  89
Baked Polenta with Spinach
  and Cheese, 140
Baked Stuffed Squash, 177
Balsamic Garlic Dressing, 79
balsamic vinegar, 59, 79
Banana Oat Muffins, 196
bananas
  Banana Oat Muffins, 196
  Fried Bananas or
    Plantains, 184
  Peach and Banana
    Flambé, 206
Barbecued Portobello
  Burgers, 161
barley, 171
  Bean and Barley Salad, 65
  Multigrain Pilaf, 176
  Mushroom Barley Soup,
    47
Basic Polenta, 141
Basic Risotto, 170
Basic Stir-fry, 117-118
Basic Vinaigrette Dressing,
  32, 77
Basic White Sauce, 107
Bean and Barley Salad, 65
beans, 10, 11
  Bean and Barley Salad,
    65
  Black Bean Soup, 51
  chick-peas. *See* chick-peas
  Cuban-Style Black Beans,
    139
  dried, 6, 53
  Gazillion Bean Salad, 72
  Homemade Refried
    Beans, 36
  lentils. *See* lentils
  as meat alternative, 20
  Muncho Grande Platter,
    37
  Pasta Fagioli, 52
  Spicy Beans and Rice,
    150
  Spicy Black Bean Dip, 27
  Sweet Potato and Pinto
    Bean Chili, 129
  Unexpectedly Delicious
    Lima Loaf, 158
  Veggie-Packed Chili,
    126-127
beets
  Sweet and Sour Roasted
    Beet Salad, 59
Biscuits From Scratch (or
  Not), 193
Black Bean Soup, 51
Bombproof Baked Macaroni
  Casserole, 106
Breaded Tofu Fingers, 157
breads
  Biscuits From Scratch (or
    Not), 193
  Fabulous Focaccia, 190
  Homemade Biscuit Mix,
    192

Jalapeño Cornbread, 191
Oatmeal Raisin Bread,
  188-189
Parmesan Onion Bread,
  194
Ridiculously Easy Cheese
  Quickbread, 195
Ultra-Quick All-Purpose
  Yeast Dough, 187
breakfast
  burrito, 26
  Fluffy Pancakes, 90
  Power-Packed Fruit
    Smoothie, 85
  Scrambled Tofu, 85
  Whole Wheat Buttermilk
    French Toast, 84
  Whole Wheat Buttermilk
    Pancakes, 91
broccoli
  Baked Broccoli Egg
    Squares, 89
  Shells Stuffed with
    Broccoli and Cheese,
    116
brown rice, 19, 169
buckwheat. See Kasha
Bulgur Pilaf, 174
bulgur wheat
  Bulgur Pilaf, 174
  as meat alternative, 19
  Taboulleh, 75
burritos
  breakfast, 26
  Full Meal Burritos, 166
buttermilk substitutes, 91

C

cabbage
  Crunchy Coleslaw, 60
  Red Cabbage with
    Apples, 179

cakes
  Amazing Eggless Dairy-
    Free Chocolate Cake,
    199
  Amazing Eggless Dairy-
    Free Orange Cake, 200
  Non-Dairy Chocolate
    Frosting, 201
  Non-Dairy Vanilla
    Frosting, 201
calcium, 16
calories, 14
Carrot Apple Muffins, 197
carrots
  Carrot Apple Muffins,
    197
  Creamy Carrot Soup, 44
  Oven-Roasted Carrot and
    Sweet Potato Casserole,
    147
  Zingy Carrot Salad, 74
Cashew Noodle Stir-fry,
  119-120
cauliflower
  Cauliflower Curry, 130
  Cream of Cauliflower
    Soup, 46
Cauliflower Curry, 130
cheese, 31
  kosher, 106
  rennet, 106
  Ridiculously Easy Cheese
    Quickbread, 195
  Salsa Cheese Bites, 33
Cheese Noodle Casserole,
  108-109
Chick-Pea and Tomato
  Soup, 42
Chick-Pea Curry, 133
chick-peas
  Chick-Pea and Tomato
    Soup, 42
  Chick-Pea Curry, 133

Hummus, 23
chili
  paste, 76
  Sweet Potato and Pinto
    Bean Chili, 129
  Veggie-Packed Chili,
    126-127
Chinese chili paste, 76
Chunky Avocado Salsa, 24
cilantro, 27
Citrus Spinach Salad, 58
Cold Zucchini Soup, 55
coriander, 27
corn, 61
  Corn and Tomato Salad,
    61
  Spicy Corn, 183
Corn and Tomato Salad, 61
Couscous Salad, 70
Cream of Cauliflower Soup,
  46
Creamy Carrot Soup, 44
Creamy Greek Dressing, 80
cremini mushrooms, 63
crepe fillings, 93
Crunchy Coleslaw, 60
Cuban-Style Black Beans,
  139
cucumbers
  Tzatziki, 28
Curried Red Lentil Soup, 50
curries
  Cauliflower Curry, 130
  Chick-Pea Curry, 133
  Fruity Raita, 131
  Potato and Pea Curry,
    132
  Veggie Raita, 131

D

dal, 185
desserts

Amazing Eggless Dairy-
Free Chocolate Cake,
199
Amazing Eggless Dairy-
Free Orange Cake, 200
Fabulous Fresh Fruit
Sorbet, 204
Fruit Compote, 205
Fruit Crisp, 202
Non-Dairy Chocolate
Frosting, 201
Non-Dairy Vanilla
Frosting, 201
Peach and Banana
Flambé, 206
Seemingly Normal
Chocolate Pudding, 203
Truly Astonishing Tofu
Chocolate Mousse, 207
vegan, 205
Dijon mustard, 57
dips
Baba Ghanouj, 29
Chunky Avocado Salsa,
24
Fresh Tomato Salsa, 26
Hummus, 23
Mexican Meltdown, 31
Spicy Black Bean Dip, 27
Tzatziki, 28
dressings
Balsamic Garlic Dressing,
79
Basic Vinaigrette
Dressing, 32, 77
Creamy Greek Dressing,
80
Incredible Oriental
Dressing, 60, 67
Sun-Dried Tomato
Vinaigrette Dressing, 78
Tofu Mayonnaise, 82

Yogurt Tahini Dressing,
81

Ė

eating out, 17, 20
eggplant
Baba Ghanouj, 29
as meat alternative, 20
Spicy Tofu and Eggplant,
121
Vegetarian Moussaka,
144-145
eggs, 10, 11
Baked Broccoli Egg
Squares, 89
Fast Frittata, 86
Quickie Quiche, 87
Tofu Egg Salad, 68
Whole Wheat Buttermilk
French Toast, 84
Zucchini and Basil Strata,
88
Eight-Vegetable Stew, 134-
135

F

Fabulous Focaccia, 190
Fabulous Fresh Fruit Sorbet,
204
Fancy French Potato Salad,
57
Fast Frittata, 86
Fluffy Pancakes, 90
freezer foods, 19
fresh foods, 19
Fresh Tomato Salsa, 26
Fried Bananas or Plantains,
184
Fried Rice with Vegetables
and Seitan or Tempeh, 124
Fruit Compote, 205

Fruit Crisp, 202
fruits, 10, 11
Fruity Raita, 131
Full Meal Burritos, 166
Fully Loaded Pasta
Primavera, 102-103

G

garam masala, 132
garlic
Roasted Garlic, 30
Tomato Garlic Green
Beans, 181
Gazillion Bean Salad, 72
ginger root, 105
Golden Vegetable Broth, 39
grains, 10, 11
barley. *See* barley
buckwheat, 175
bulgur wheat. *See* bulgur
wheat
Couscous Salad, 70
Kasha, 175
millet, 171
Multigrain Pilaf, 176
quinoa, 171
rice. *See* rice
Spicy Vegetable
Couscous, 136-137
Green and White Lasagne,
112-113
green beans
Tomato Garlic Green
Beans, 181
Green Salad, 58
Grillable Tofu Veggie
Burgers, 162-163

H

helpful hints, 15

Homemade Biscuit Mix, 192
Homemade Refried Beans, 36
Hummus, 23

i

imitation meat, 20
Incredible Onion Tart, 146
Incredible Oriental Dressing, 60, 67
Indian Vegetable Pilaf, 151
iron, 15

J

Jalapeño Cornbread, 126, 191

K

Kasha, 175
kosher cheese, 106

L

labels, 160
lacto-ovo vegetarian, 10
lacto-vegetarian, 10
lasagne
    Green and White Lasagne, 112-113
    Multivegetable Lasagne, 110-111
legumes. See beans
Lemon Rice, 172
Lentil Dal, 185
lentils
    Curried Red Lentil Soup, 50
    Lentil Dal, 185

as meat alternative, 19
Quick Lentil Soup, 43
Veggie Paté, 32
lima beans, 158

M

Mexican Meltdown, 31
Mexican Red Rice, 173
milk, 10, 11
milk alternatives, 10, 11
millet, 171
moussaka, 144-145
muffins
    Banana Oat Muffins, 196
    Carrot Apple Muffins, 197
Multigrain Pilaf, 176
Multivegetable Lasagne, 110-111
Muncho Grande Platter, 37
mung bean sprouts, 118
Mushroom Barley Soup, 47
Mushroom Stroganoff with Seitan (or Not), 138
mushrooms, 63
    Barbecued Portobello Burgers, 161
    cremini mushrooms, 63
    as meat alternative, 20
    Mushroom Barley Soup, 47
    Mushroom Stroganoff with Seitan (or Not), 138
    No-Brainer Mushroom Alfredo, 101
    oyster mushrooms, 63
    portobello mushrooms, 63
    shiitake mushrooms, 63
    Stuffed Portobello Mushrooms, 159

Warm Mushroom Salad, 62-63
white button mushrooms, 63
mustard, 57

N

Nearly Normal Shepherd's Pie, 142-143
No-Brainer Mushroom Alfredo, 101
Non-Dairy Chocolate Frosting, 201
Non-Dairy Vanilla Frosting, 201
noodles. See pasta and noodles

O

Oatmeal Raisin Bread, 188-189
occasional vegetarian, 10
Old-Fashioned Potato Soup, 45
olive oil, 78
onions, 137
    Incredible Onion Tart, 146
    Orange and Red Onion Salad, 64
    Pizza with Sweet and Sour Caramelized Onions, 155
Orange and Red Onion Salad, 64
oranges, 64
osteoporosis, 16
Oven-Roasted Carrot and Sweet Potato Casserole, 147

Oven-Roasted Vegetables, 181
ovo-vegetarian, 10
oyster mushrooms, 63

P

Pad Thai, 122-123
pancakes
    Fluffy Pancakes, 90
    Plain Crepes, 92-93
    Whole Wheat Buttermilk Pancakes, 91
pantry staples, 18
Parmesan Onion Bread, 194
Pasta à la Caprese, 104
pasta and noodles
    All-Purpose Tomato Pasta Sauce, 95-96
    Bombproof Baked Macaroni Casserole, 106
    Cashew Noodle Stir-fry, 119-120
    Cheese Noodle Casserole, 108-109
    Couscous Salad, 70
    freezing, 101
    Fully Loaded Pasta Primavera, 102-103
    Green and White Lasagne, 112-113
    macaroni, 103
    Multivegetable Lasagne, 110-111
    No-Brainer Mushroom Alfredo, 101
    one serving, 103
    Pad Thai, 122-123
    Pasta à la Caprese, 104
    Pasta Puttanesca, 100
    Pasta Salad, 71
    Pasta with Sun-Dried Tomatoes, 99

Peculiar Peanut Pasta, 105
    Roasted Tomato Fettuccine, 98
    Shells Stuffed with Broccoli and Cheese, 116
    Simple Sesame Noodle Salad, 67
    Spicy Vegetable Couscous, 136-137
    vegan alert, 103
Pasta Fagioli, 52
Pasta Puttanesca, 100
Pasta Salad, 71
Pasta with Sun-Dried Tomatoes, 99
Peach and Banana Flambé, 206
Peculiar Peanut Pasta, 105
Perfect Pesto Sauce, 97
Phenomenal Minestrone Soup, 48-49
phyllo pastry, 148
pilaf
    Bulgur Pilaf, 174
    Indian Vegetable Pilaf, 151
    Multigrain Pilaf, 176
pizza topping ideas, 153
Pizza with Pesto, Goat Cheese and Sun-Dried Tomatoes, 151
Pizza with Sweet and Sour Caramelized Onions, 155
Pizza with Tomato Sauce and Whatever, 152
Plain Crepes, 92-93
polenta
    Baked Polenta with Spinach and Cheese, 140
    Basic Polenta, 141

sliceable, 141
portobello mushrooms, 63
    Barbecued Portobello Burgers, 161
    Stuffed Portobello Mushrooms, 159
Potato and Pea Curry, 132
Potato Kugel, 182
potatoes
    Fancy French Potato Salad, 57
    Nearly Normal Shepherd's Pie, 142-143
    Old-Fashioned Potato Soup, 45
    Potato and Pea Curry, 132
    Potato Kugel, 182
Power-Packed Fruit Smoothie, 85
protein, 14-15
Pseudo-Hollandaise Sauce, 32, 111

Q

Quesadillas, 35
quiche, 87
Quick Lentil Soup, 43
Quickie Quiche, 87
quinoa, 171

R

raita
    Fruity Raita, 131
    Veggie Raita, 131
Ratatouille, 178
recipe adaptations, 20-21
Red Cabbage with Apples, 179
red peppers, 153

Red Star™ nutritional yeast, 14
Refried Beans, 36
rennet, 106
riboflavin, 16
rice
    basic risotto, 170
    brown rice, 169
    cooking basics, 168-169
    Fried Rice with Vegetables and Seitan or Tempeh, 124
    Indian Vegetable Pilaf, 151
    Lemon Rice, 172
    Mexican Red Rice, 173
    Multigrain Pilaf, 176
    Spicy Beans and Rice, 150
    white rice, 168
    Wild and Brown Rice Salad, 73
    wild rice, 169
Ridiculously Easy Cheese Quickbread, 195
Roasted Garlic, 30
roasted red peppers, 153
Roasted Tomato Fettuccine, 98
Roasted Veggie Variation (Broth), 40

§

salads
    Authentic Greek Salad, 66
    Bean and Barley Salad, 65
    Citrus Spinach Salad, 58
    Corn and Tomato Salad, 61
    Couscous Salad, 70
    Crunchy Coleslaw, 60
    Fancy French Potato Salad, 57
    Gazillion Bean Salad, 72
    Green Salad, 58
    Orange and Red Onion Salad, 64
    Pasta Salad, 71
    Simple Sesame Noodle Salad, 67
    Spicy Oriental Asparagus Salad, 76
    Sweet and Sour Roasted Beet Salad, 59
    Tabboulleh, 75
    Tofu Egg Salad, 68
    Warm Mushroom Salad, 62-63
    Wild and Brown Rice Salad, 73
    Zingy Carrot Salad, 74
salsa
    Chunky Avocado Salsa, 24
    Fresh Tomato Salsa, 26
    Salsa Cheese Bites, 33
sauces
    All-Purpose Tomato Pasta Sauce, 95-96
    Basic White Sauce, 107
    Perfect Pesto Sauce, 97
    Pseudo-Hollandaise Sauce, 32, 111
Scrambled Tofu, 85
Seemingly Normal Chocolate Pudding, 203
seitan, 18, 125
    Fried Rice with Vegetables and Seitan or Tempeh, 124
    Mushroom Stroganoff with Seitan (or Not), 138
sesame oil, 121
Shells Stuffed with Broccoli and Cheese, 116
Shepherd's Pie, 142-143
shiitake mushrooms, 63
side dishes
    Fried Bananas or Plantains, 184
    Lentil Dal, 185
    Oven-Roasted Vegetables, 181
    Potato Kugel, 182
    Ratatouille, 178
    Red Cabbage with Apples, 179
    Spicy Corn, 183
    Tomato Garlic Green Beans, 181
Simple Sesame Noodle Salad, 67
snacks. See appetizers
soups
    African Peanut Soup, 54
    Black Bean Soup, 51
    Chick-Pea and Tomato Soup, 42
    Cold Zucchini Soup, 55
    Cream of Cauliflower Soup, 46
    Creamy Carrot Soup, 44
    Curried Red Lentil Soup, 50
    Golden Vegetable Broth, 39
    Mushroom Barley Soup, 47
    Old-Fashioned Potato Soup, 45
    Pasta Fagioli, 52
    Phenomenal Minestrone Soup, 48-49
    Quick Lentil Soup, 43
    Roasted Veggie Variation

(Broth), 40
Split Pea Soup, 41
stock bag, 40
soy cheese, 19, 109
soy milk, 19, 109, 205
Spanakopita, 148-149
spices, 164
Spicy Beans and Rice, 150
Spicy Black Bean Dip, 27
Spicy Corn, 183
Spicy Oriental Asparagus
Salad, 76
Spicy Tofu and Eggplant,
121
Spicy Vegetable Couscous,
136-137
spinach
Citrus Spinach Salad, 58
Spanakopita, 148-149
split cooking, 114-115
Split Pea Soup, 41
sprouts, 118, 120
squash, 177
starters. *See* appetizers
stew, 134-135
stir-fry
Basic Stir-fry, 117-118
Cashew Noodle Stir-fry,
119-120
stock bag, 40
Stuffed Portobello
Mushrooms, 159
Sun-Dried Tomato
Vinaigrette Dressing, 78
supplies, 16-17
Sweet and Sour Roasted
Beet Salad, 59
Sweet Potato and Pinto Bean
Chili, 129
sweet potatoes, 128
Oven-Roasted Carrot and
Sweet Potato Casserole,
147

Sweet Potato and Pinto
Bean Chili, 129

T

Taboulleh, 75
tahini, 22, 81
tempeh, 18, 165
Fried Rice with
Vegetables and Seitan or
Tempeh, 124
Teriyaki Tempeh Kabobs,
164
Teriyaki Tempeh Kabobs,
164
texturized vegetable protein.
See TVP
tofu, 69
Baked Barbecue Tofu
Steaks, 156
Breaded Tofu Fingers,
157
frozen and defrosted, 18
Grillable Tofu Veggie
Burgers, 162-163
Scrambled Tofu, 85
Spicy Tofu and Eggplant,
121
Tofu Egg Salad, 68
Tofu Mayonnaise, 82
Truly Astonishing Tofu
Chocolate Mousse, 207
Tofu Egg Salad, 68
Tofu Mayonnaise, 82
Tomato Garlic Green Beans,
181
tomatoes, 96
All-Pupose Tomato Pasta
Sauce, 95-96
Authentic Greek Salad,
66
Chick-Pea and Tomato
Soup, 42

Corn and Tomato Salad,
61
Fresh Tomato Salsa, 26
Mexican Meltdown, 31
Pasta à la Caprese, 104
Pasta with Sun-Dried
Tomatoes, 99
Pizza with Pesto, Goat
Cheese and Sun-Dried
Tomatoes, 151
Ratatoutille, 178
Roasted Tomato
Fettuccine, 98
Tomato Garlic Green
Beans, 181
Truly Astonishing Tofu
Chocolate Mousse, 207
TVP, 20, 143
Tzatziki, 28

U

Ultra-Quick All-Purpose
Yeast Dough, 187
Unexpectedly Delicious
Lima Loaf, 158

V

vegan, 10, 103
vegetable broth, 18, 39, 42
vegetables, 10, 11
vegetarian food guide, 12-13
Vegetarian Moussaka, 144-
145
Veggie Paté, 32
Veggie Pot Pie, 135
Veggie Raita, 131
Veggie-Packed Chili, 126-
127
vitamin B-12, 16
vitamin C, 15
vitamin D, 16

W

Warm Mushroom Salad, 62
wheat gluten. *See* seitan
white button mushrooms,
  63
white rice, 169
  see also rice
Whole Wheat Buttermilk
  French Toast, 84
Whole Wheat Buttermilk
  Pancakes, 91
Wild and Brown Rice Salad,
  73
wild rice, 169
  see also rice

Y

Yogurt Tahini Dressing, 81
yogurt
  Veggie Raita, 131
  Fruity Raita, 131

Z

zinc, 16
Zingy Carrot Salad, 74
zucchini
  Cold Zucchini Soup, 55
  Zucchini and Basil Strata,
    88
  Zucchini Appetizers, 34
Zucchini and Basil Strata,
  88
Zucchini Appetizers, 34